Regenerative Medicine for Peripheral Artery Disease

Regenerative Medicine for Peripheral Artery Disease

Edited by

Emile R. Mohler III

Perelman School of Medicine
at the University of Pennsylvania
Division of Cardiovascular Medicine
Department of Medicine
Philadelphia, PA, United States

Brian H. Annex

University of Virginia
Division of Cardiovascular Medicine
Department of Medicine
Charlottesville, VA, United States

ELSEVIER

AMSTERDAM • BOSTON • HEIDELBERG • LONDON
NEW YORK • OXFORD • PARIS • SAN DIEGO
SAN FRANCISCO • SINGAPORE • SYDNEY • TOKYO
Academic Press is an imprint of Elsevier

AP

Academic Press is an imprint of Elsevier
125 London Wall, London EC2Y 5AS, United Kingdom
525 B Street, Suite 1800, San Diego, CA 92101-4495, United States
50 Hampshire Street, 5th Floor, Cambridge, MA 02139, United States
The Boulevard, Langford Lane, Kidlington, Oxford OX5 1GB, UK

British Library Cataloguing-in-Publication Data

A catalogue record for this book is available from the British Library

Library of Congress Cataloging-in-Publication Data

A catalog record for this book is available from the Library of Congress

ISBN: 978-0-12-801344-1

Publisher: Mica Haley
Acquisition Editor: Stacy Masucci
Editorial Project Manager: Sam Young
Production Project Manager: Julia Haynes
Designer: Matt Limbert

Typeset by Thomson Digital

To our families for their patience and support for this endeavor, and to our patients, for whom we continue to strive for better lives.

E.R. Mohler III, MD
B.H. Annex, MD

Contents

List of Contributors

Numbers in Parentheses indicate the pages on which the author's contributions begin.

B.H. Annex (1), University of Virginia, Division of Cardiovascular Medicine, Department of Medicine, Charlottesville, VA, United States

T. Asahara (71), Department of Regenerative Medicine Science, Tokai University School of Medicine, Isehara, Kanagawa, Japan

M.Y. Flugelman (91), Perelman School of Medicine at the University of Pennsylvania, Division of Cardiovascular Medicine, Department of Medicine, Philadelphia, PA, United States

S. Hazarika (1), University of Virginia, Division of Cardiovascular Medicine, Department of Medicine, Charlottesville, VA, United States

M. Ii (71), Department of Pharmacology, Group of Translational Stem Cell Research, Osaka Medical College, Takatsuki, Osaka, Japan

W.S. Jones (117), Department of Medicine, Duke University Medical Center, Durham, NC, United States

A. Kawamoto (71), Unit of Regenerative Medicine, Institute of Biomedical Research and Innovation, Chuo-ku, Kobe, Japan

D. Kopin (117), Department of Medicine, Duke University Medical Center, Durham, NC, United States

C.M. Kramer (95), Departments of Medicine, Radiology and Medical Imaging, and the Cardiovascular Imaging Center, University of Virginia Health System, Charlottesville, VA and the Knight Cardiovascular Institute, Oregon Health & Science University, Portland, OR, United States

J.R. Lindner (95), Departments of Medicine, Radiology and Medical Imaging, and the Cardiovascular Imaging Center, University of Virginia Health System, Charlottesville, VA and the Knight Cardiovascular Institute, Oregon Health & Science University, Portland, OR, United States

K.L. March (27), Indiana Center for Vascular Biology and Medicine (ICVBM); Department of Medicine, Richard L. Roudebush VA Center for Regenerative Medicine; Krannert Institute of Cardiology, Indianapolis, IN, United States

W. Marston (137), University of North Carolina, School of Medicine, Division of Vascular Surgery, Department of Surgery, Chapel Hill, NC, United States

H. Masuda (71), Department of Regenerative Medicine Science, Tokai University School of Medicine, Isehara, Kanagawa, Japan

E.R. Mohler III (17, 91), Perelman School of Medicine at the University of Pennsylvania, Division of Cardiovascular Medicine, Department of Medicine, Philadelphia, PA, United States

M.P. Murphy (27), Indiana Center for Vascular Biology and Medicine (ICVBM); Department of Medicine, Richard L. Roudebush VA Center for Regenerative Medicine; Department of Surgery, Indiana University Center for Aortic Disease (IU-CAD); Indiana University Department of Surgery (IUSM), Indianapolis, IN, United States

T.J. Povsic (43), Duke Clinical Research Institute, Duke Medicine, Durham, NC, United States

A.M. Sharma (1), University of Virginia, Division of Cardiovascular Medicine, Department of Medicine, Charlottesville, VA, United States

J. Solanki (1), University of Virginia, Division of Cardiovascular Medicine, Department of Medicine, Charlottesville, VA, United States

K.S. Telukuntla (17, 91), Perelman School of Medicine at the University of Pennsylvania, Division of Cardiovascular Medicine, Department of Medicine, Philadelphia, PA, United States

J. Xie (27), Indiana Center for Vascular Biology and Medicine (ICVBM); Department of Medicine, Richard L. Roudebush VA Center for Regenerative Medicine; Indiana University Department of Surgery (IUSM), Indianapolis, IN, United States

M. Yadava (95), Departments of Medicine, Radiology and Medical Imaging, and the Cardiovascular Imaging Center, University of Virginia Health System, Charlottesville, VA and the Knight Cardiovascular Institute, Oregon Health & Science University, Portland, OR, United States

Preface

Peripheral artery disease (PAD) is a prevalent disease and frequently manifests with symptoms of claudication. This results in severe impairment of quality of life and may ultimately lead to amputation. The treatment of PAD continues to evolve, but it is fundamentally focused on improvement in exercise performance and control of risk factors and methods to improve claudication symptoms. The current treatment options for claudication include a supervised exercise program, with or without cilostazol, or revascularization techniques. However, due to limitations of medical management and revascularization, there is a need for a cell therapy approach to promote limb angiogenesis and collateral development in order to improve claudication symptoms.

The primary objective of *Regenerative Medicine for Peripheral Artery Disease* is to provide the reader with the most current information on various regenerative approaches for claudication. The text is unique in that it covers a broad range of published clinical studies demonstrating novel cell-based strategies to improve claudication symptoms or save the leg in the setting of critical limb ischemia. In addition, an interactive web site is available through Elsevier Publishing Company which includes detailed references and continued medical education for this topic.

This reference was designed to provide an easy-to-use resource for people interested in the history of and latest regenerative approaches for PAD. We hope that ultimately one day a regenerative therapeutic approach will emerge and result in better care for our patients.

E.R. Mohler III, MD
B.H. Annex, MD

Chapter 1

Angiogenesis in Peripheral Artery Disease: Focus on Growth Factor Therapy

A.M. Sharma, MBBS, S. Hazarika, MD, J. Solanki, BS, B.H. Annex, MD
University of Virginia, Division of Cardiovascular Medicine, Department of Medicine, Charlottesville, VA, United States

INTRODUCTION

Lower extremity peripheral artery disease (PAD) is narrowing or occlusion of the lower extremity arteries primarily due to atherosclerosis (Fig. 1.1). It is typically diagnosed in the vascular laboratory by an abnormally low ankle–brachial index (ABI) study which is the ratio of highest blood pressure in the ankle arteries (dorsalis pedis or posterior tibialis) and the highest blood pressure in the brachial arteries. The clinical manifestations of PAD range from asymptomatic disease to intermittent claudication to critical limb ischemia (CLI) depending on the degree of reduction in blood flow to the extremities. Intermittent claudication (IC) is when one experiences pain or cramping with exertion in the lower extremity that is relieved with rest. CLI is the most aggressive form of PAD presenting as rest pain or nonhealing ulcers and/or gangrene of the lower extremities, often resulting in amputation [1]. PAD particularly CLI has a very high mortality especially due to cardiovascular causes [1]. Although PAD has be underdiagnosed and underrecognized for a long time, it is now gaining significant recognition in the medical and general community as it is estimated to be present in up to 8–12 million people in USA itself and up to 20% of the population above the age of 65 years may have PAD [2].

Risk factors for PAD are similar to any atherosclerotic disease as noted in Table 1.1 [1]. It is now well established that atherosclerotic plaque formation in the arteries is an inflammatory condition which is often initiated by a combination of genetic and environmental factors. The various stages of atherosclerosis are noted in Table 1.2 [3]. Management with statins, antiplatelet, and angiotensin convertase enzyme inhibitors provides a benefit in preventing disease progression and reducing morbidity and mortality related to cardiac causes; however, the primary therapeutic goal to restore blood flow to the skeletal muscle

Regenerative Medicine for Peripheral Artery Disease. http://dx.doi.org/10.1016/B978-0-12-801344-1.00001-2

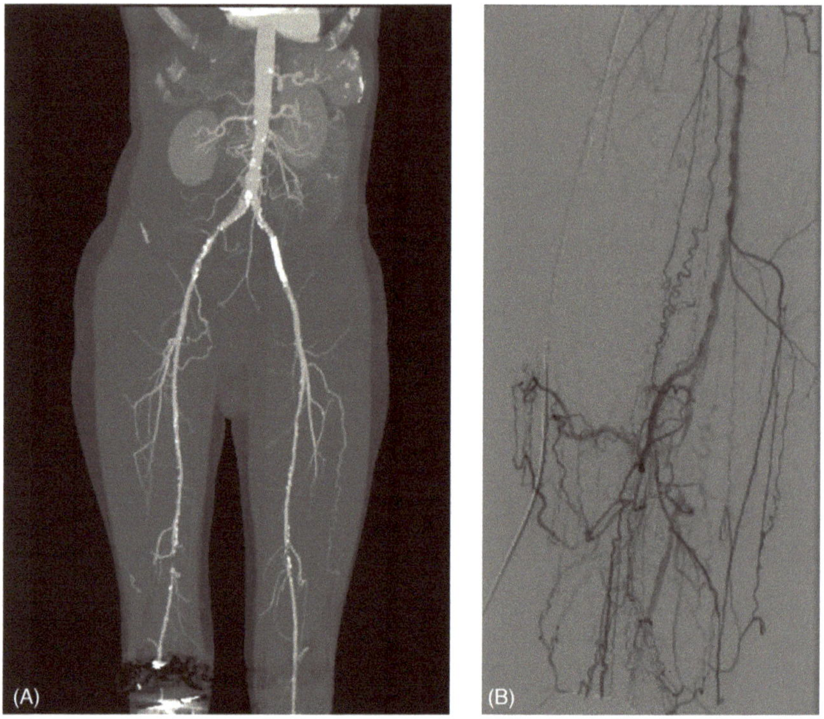

FIGURE 1.1 A 6-year-old man with intermittent claudication. A shows CT angiogram of the abdominal aortal with ileofemoral runoff shows a short segment occlusion of the superficial femoral artery bilaterally with moderate atherosclerosis bilaterally in the iliac arteries. Patent external iliac stent in the left common iliac artery. B shows short segment occlusion of the right superficial femoral artery with collateralization.

TABLE 1.1 Risk Factors for Lower Extremity PAD

1. Cigarette smoking
2. Diabetes mellitus
3. Hypertension
4. Dyslipidemia
5. Elevated inflammatory markers (hs-CRP)
6. Hyperhomocysteinemia
7. Elevated fibrinogen level

PAD, peripheral artery disease; *hs-CRP*, high sensitivity C-reactive protein.

beyond the area of occlusion for treating IC or CLI is not achieved through medical management. Currently, therapeutic options for treatment of symptomatic PAD consist mainly of endovascular or surgical techniques which are not always effective in treating symptoms or preventing amputations. Often relief is not achieved adequately even with successful revascularization, outcomes of

TABLE 1.2 Stages of Atherosclerosis

Migration of leukocytes from the blood to the intima
↓
Maturation of the monocyte into macrophages and their conversion to foam cells with lipid intake
↓
Migration and proliferation of the smooth muscle cells (SMCs) in the intima.
↓
Plaque macrophage and SMC apoptosis, leading to formation of lipid rich necrotic core plaques.
↓
Rupture of lipid rich necrotic core plaques
↓
Exposure of tissue components from the ruptured plaque to the coagulation factors in the blood
↓
Thrombosis in the arteries causing severe narrowing or occlusion often leads to tissue ischemia

amputations or symptoms because of delayed complications related to these procedures such as stent restenosis or stent/graft thrombosis as well as due to inability to revasularize distal vessels. Due to lack of definitive therapy, medical or otherwise, in the treatment of symptomatic PAD there is a need to develop strategies to promote neovascularization which often requires a combination of angiogenesis, arteriogenesis, and vasculogenesis. Angiogenesis is the process of formation of new capillaries from preexisting vessels. These capillaries are up to 12 μm in diameter and typically lack well-developed tunica media [4]. Neorevascularization through arteriogenesis have larger vessels (20–100 μm in diameter) with fully developed tunica media, whereas vasculogenesis is in situ formation of blood vessels [5,6].

Therapeutic angiogenesis is a promising strategy to treat PAD particularly CLI. Although its clinical utility in PAD has not been established yet, there has been significant progress in this field in the last five decades since its first observation by Judah Folkman in 1971 in a tumor [7]. Tissue ischemia is the most potent stimulator for angiogenesis in vivo. Hypoxia inducible factor-1 (HIF-1α) is a key transcription factor that is stabilized under conditions of tissue ischemia [8]. HIF-1α stimulates transcription of several key angiogenic growth factors and growth factor receptors, including vascular endothelial growth factor (VEGF-A) [9]. In response to a coordinated process between growth factors, growth factor receptors, several adhesion molecules, and tissue matrix metalloproteinases, endothelial cells proliferate, invaginate, migrate, and form new capillaries [10]. Therapeutic angiogenesis is a strategy to utilize this physiological process to enhance formation of new vasculature distal to the site of an arterial occlusion. A promising area of therapeutic angiogenesis is cell therapy. Embryonic stem cells or adult pluripotent cells have the potential to differentiate into desired cell types on the basis of the cellular microenvironments. In addition to homing to ischemic tissue and maturing into specific cell types, cell therapy can also produce arrays of cytokines/growth factors that can have endocrine and paracrine effects, thereby leading to a more sustained proangiogenic milieu.

GROWTH FACTOR THERAPY IN PERIPHERAL ARTERY DISEASE

Therapeutic angiogenesis has mostly been targeted in CLI with no revascularization options. In an attempt to induce therapeutic angiogenesis in ischemic tissue, several different approaches have been under investigation. Initial studies investigated effects of direct injection of recombinant growth-factor proteins into the ischemic tissue. However, these studies met with significant limitations, including ineffective delivery and lack of homogenous uptake by tissues as well as limited bioavailability of injected growth factors due to their short half-lives.

Since then, studies have evolved to investigate delivery of growth factors using different gene therapy strategies, including viral and nonviral vectors, naked and plasmid DNA which are discussed in great detail in the chapter. Numerous growth factors have now been studied in the treatment of PAD especially fibroblast growth factor (FGF), vascular endothelial growth factor (VEGF), and hepatocyte growth factor (HGF) being commonly evaluated (Table 1.3).

FIBROBLAST GROWTH FACTOR

FGF are heparin-binding growth factors consisting of 22 proteins with similar structures [11]. They are key players in proliferation and differentiation of cells and tissues [12]. Since four receptor subtypes can be activated by 20 different FGF ligands, they function as pluripotent growth factors and so far, FGF-1, FGF-2, and FGF-4 have been strongly implicated in angiogenesis [13,14].

The first phase-I clinical trial using FGF therapy for PAD with IC was published in 2000 by Lazarous et al. [15]. In this double-blind, placebo-controlled dose-escalation trial, IC patients with an ABI < 0.8 were delivered through

TABLE 1.3 Human Clinical Trials of Growth Factor Therapy in Peripheral Artery Disease

Author (year)	Growth factor	Study phase and type	PAD type	Delivery route	Number of subjects	Vector	Results
Lazarous (2000)	FGF	I RCT, placebo, double blind	IC	IA	15	None	Increased calf blood flow
Lederman (2002)	FGF	II RCT	IC	IA	190	None	Increased PWT
Comerota (2002)	FGF	I	CLI	IM	51	Naked plasmid	No AE; decreased rest pain, ulcer size, and improved $TcPO_2$
Marui (2007)	FGF	I-IIa	CLI	IM	7	Gelatin hydrogel	Increased distance walked, $TCPO_2$, ulcer healing. Decreased rest pain. ABI unchanged
Nikol (2008)	FGF	II	CLI	IM	125	Naked plasmid	No difference in ulcer healing; lower amputation rates
Hashimoto (2009)	FGF	I	CLI	IM	8	Gelatin hydrogel	No AE
Belch (2011)	FGF	III	CLI	IM	525	Naked plasmid	No difference in amputations or mortality
Takagi (2011)	FGF	II	CLI	IM	25	Gelatin hydrogel	Decreased rest pain and improved $TcPO_2$
Kamugai (2015)	FGF	I-IIa	CLI	IM	10	Gelatin hydrogel	Increased $TcPO_2$ and distance walked
Isner (1996)	VEGF 165	I	CLI	IA	1	Naked plasmid	Increased collaterals

(Continued)

TABLE 1.3 Human Clinical Trials of Growth Factor Therapy in Peripheral Artery Disease (*cont.*)

Author (year)	Growth factor	Study phase and type	PAD type	Delivery route	Number of subjects	Vector	Results
Baumgartner (1998)	VEGF 165	I	CLI	IM	9	Naked plasmid	Increased ABI, vascularity, ulcer healing, and distal flow
Simovic (2001)	VEGF 165	I	CLI	IM	17	Naked plasmid	Increased ABI and symptom scores
Shyu (2003)	VEGF 165	I	CLI	IM	21	Naked plasmid	Increased ABI, distal circulation, and ulcer healing; decreased rest pain
Kusumanto (2006)	VEGF 165	II RCT, placebo controlled, double blind	CLI	IM	54	Naked plasmid	No difference in amputations, increased hemodynamics, ulcer healing, pain relief
Mohler (2003)	VEGF	I	CLI	IM	18	DNA	No AE
Makinen (2002)	VEGF 165	II RCT, placebo controlled, double blind	CLI	IA	37	Naked plasmid or adenovirus	Increased vascularity No difference in Rutherford class, ABI, major amputations, ulcer healing, rest pain
Rajagopalan (2003)	VEGF 121	II Double blind, placebo controlled, RCT	IC	IM	105	Adenovirus	No difference in PWT or claudication onset time, ABI or QOL
Muona (2012)	VEGF	Phase II	CLI	IM	54	Adenovirus or naked plasmid	No difference in AE compared to placebo in 10 years
Morishita (2004)	HGF	I	CLI	IM	6		Improvement in rest pain, ABI, and ulcer healing

Powell (2008)	HGF	Phase I/II placebo, double blind	CLI	IM	104	Naked plasmid	No difference in safety, ABI/TBI, major amputations, ulcer healing; improvement in $TcPO_2$ in high dose group
Powell (2010)	HGF	Phase II RCT, placebo	CLI	IM	27	Naked plasmid	Improvement in TBI, pain symptoms; no difference in ulcer healing, major amputations, and mortality
Shigematsu (2010)	HGF	III	CLI	IM	44	Naked plasmid	Decreased rest pain and ulcer size, no difference in ABI, amps; improvement in QoL, Rutherford score
Gu (2011)	HGF	I	CLI	IM	21	Naked plasmid	Improvement in ABI, pain, $TcPO_2$, and ulcer healing
Cui (2015)	HGF	I	CLI	IM	21	Naked plasmid	Improvement in ABI, rest pain, $TcPO_2$, and ulcer healing
Makino (2012)	HGF	I/IIa	IC	IM	22	Naked plasmid	Improvement in ABI, rest pain, and ulcer healing
Rajagopalan (2007)	HIF-1a	phase I: RCT, double blind, placebo	CLI	IM	34	Adenovirus	No difference in safety and improved rest pain, ulcer healing, and ABI
Creager (2011)	HIF-1a	III double-blinded RCT	IC	IM	289	Adenovirus	No difference in PWT, claudication onset time, ABI, or QoL

FGF, fibroblast growth factor; *IC*, intermittent claudication; *RCT*, randomized controlled trial; *incr.*, increased; *AE*, adverse events; *decr.*, decreased; *$TcPO_2$*, transcutaneous oxygen pressure; *VEGF*, vascular endothelial growth factor; *PWT*, peak walking time; *QOL*, quality of life; *HGF*, hepatocyte growth factor; *HIF-1a*, hypoxia-induced factor-1 alfa.

femoral artery, a placebo or basic FGF (bFGF) at doses of 10 once, 30 or 30 μg/kg on 2 consecutive days. The primary objective of this study was safety and efficacy of bFGF. At various points over 12 months, retinal photography and plethysmography were performed. Results were promising and reported increased calf blood flow by 66 ± 26% at 1 month and by 153 ± 51% at 6 months in bFGF-treated patients ($n = 9$, $p = 0.002$) with no change in placebo group. It was concluded that intraarterial bFGF was safe and it even increased calf blood flow. Later on recombinant FGF (rFGF) was evaluated in the TRAFFIC study in which 190 patients with IC were randomized to either placebo on days 1 and 30 ($n = 63$); rFGF-2 (30 microg/kg) on day 1 and placebo on day 30 (single-dose, $n = 66$); or rFGF-2 (30 microg/kg) on days 1 and 30 (double dose, $n = 61$) [16]. Of the 174 patients present in the study at 90 days, peak walking time (PWT) increased by 0.60 in placebo versus 1.77 min in single dose and 1.54 min in double-dose rFGF, thereby indicating clinical benefit with use of FGF-2. In 2002, the first phase-I clinical trial in CLI subjects was performed by Comerota et al. They evaluated the safety and tolerability of a naked plasmid vector encoding FGF-1 (NV1FGF) administered intramuscularly to the ischemic limbs of 51 CLI patients [17]. Sixty-six adverse events were reported; however none were related to study drug directly. Secondary endpoints showed a reduction in rest pain ($p < 0.001$), reduction in ulcer size ($p < 0.01$), and improved $TCPO_2$ ($p < 0.01$). In 2007, Marui et al pursued a phase-I–IIa trial in 7 patients with CLI to evaluate the efficacy of a sustained release bFGF injected into the gastrocnemius using a gelatin hydrogel [18]. At 4 and 24 weeks, safety and feasibility were evaluated and significant improvements were observed in the distance walked in 6 min (295 ± 42 m vs 491 ± 85 m for pretreatment vs after 24 weeks, $p = 0.023$) and in transcutaneous oxygen pressure ($TcPO_2$) (53.5 ± 5.2 mmHg vs 65.5 ± 4.0 mmHg, $p = 0.03$). Rest pain was also better (3.5 ± 0.2 vs 1.0 ± 0.6, $p = 0.022$) although ABI were unchanged. Five patients had a nonhealing foot ulcer, of which ulcer healed completely in three, partially in one and remained the same in one patient. In 2008, another phase-II clinical trial in CLI patients randomizing 125 CLI patients with no revascularization options to either placebo or NV1FGF administered IM [19]. The primary endpoint of complete healing of at least one ulcer at 25 weeks with NV1FGF use was similar to placebo (19.6% vs 14.3%; $p = 0.514$) but the risk of all amputations [hazard ratio (HR) 0.498; $p = 0.015$] and major amputations (HR 0.371; $p = 0.015$) was lower with NV1FGF use. In 2009, Hashimoto et al. conducted a nonrandomized trial to evaluate safety and efficacy of 100 μg of bFGF using gelatin hydrogel suspension in eight CLI patients with no adverse and some improvements in symptoms [20]. Later, on a phase-III trial (TAMARIS), randomizing 525 CLI patients unsuitable for revascularization to placebo or NV1FGF1 delivered IM [21]. Unfortunately the primary endpoint of major amputation or death was similar in NV1FGF and placebo group (33% vs 36%; HR 1.11, 95% CI 0.83 – 1.49; $p = 0.48$). Another study published in 2011 by Takagi et al. randomized patients with PAD to receive injectable gelatin hydrogel with either b-FGF or autologous bone marrow mononuclear cell implantation (BMCI) [22]. At

4 weeks follow-up, both groups had similar results with significant improvements in visual analog pain scale (VAS) (b-FGF 67 ± 15 to 4 ± 5, $p < 0.01$, BMCI 67 ± 42 to 5 ± 9 mm, $p < 0.01$) and $TcPO_2$ (b-FGF 16 ± 14 to 47 ± 17, $p < 0.01$, BMCI 13 ± 13 to 37 ± 21 mmHg, $p < 0.01$) and no changes in (99m) technetium−tetrofosmin, ankle−brachial index, and 2-year predicted prognosis. Most recently in 2015, Kamugai et al. published their results of sustained release bFGF using gelatin hydrogels in CLI patients [23]. In this phase-I−IIa study, 10 CLI patients were injected with 200 μg of bFGF intramuscularly (IM) in the ischemic limb. At 24 weeks, $TcPO_2$ improved significantly (28.4 ± 8.4 vs 46.2 ± 13.0 mmHg for pretreatment vs after 24 weeks, $p < 0.01$) as well the secondary endpoints of distance walked in 6 min (255 ± 105 vs 318 ± 127 m, $p = 0.02$), Rutherford classification (4.4 ± 0.5 vs 3.1 ± 1.4, $p = 0.02$), rest pain scale (1.7 ± 1.0 vs 1.2 ± 1.3, $p = 0.03$), and the cyanotic scale (2.0 ± 1.1 vs 0.9 ± 0.9, $p < 0.01$) showed statistically significant improvement with no safety concerns.

VASCULAR ENDOTHELIAL GROWTH FACTOR

The vascular endothelial growth factor (VEGF) group of cytokines has been extensively studied and consists of VEGF-A, VEGF-B, VEGF-C, VEGF-D, VEGF-E, and placenta growth factor (PGF). Of these, VEGF-A plays a key role in angiogenic activity by stimulating migration of endothelial cells, encouraging matrix metalloproteinase activity, creating blood vessel lumen, and acting as a chemotactic marker for macrophages and granulocytes. Furthermore, VEGF-A is a vasodilator and increases vascular permeability. Not all VEGF-A have angiogenic activity, in fact there is an antiangiogenic form too [24]. VEGF-A is also notable for its isoforms of which VEGF121, 121b, 145, 165, 165b, 189, and 206 are present in humans. VEGF-B is involved in embryonic angiogenesis and VEGF-C and VEGF-D are more concerned with angiogenesis in the lymphatic system [25]. The VEGF receptors are tyrosine kinase molecules, leading to dimerization and activation through transphosphorylation. When a tissue is ischemic, it releases HIF, which encourages the release and migration of VEGF-A which can bind to its receptors on endothelial cells and initiate angiogenesis [26]. Interestingly, certain type of VEGF has also been implicated in contributing to metastasis or cancer development [24]. VEGF 121 and VEGF 165 which do not bind to heparin and are primarily found in circulation have frequently been evaluated in PAD-related clinical studies [25,27]. Initial animal model studies showed great promise with VEGF therapy which led to human trials [28–30]. The first case of VEGF therapy in humans for CLI was reported by Isner et al. in which a 71-year-old CLI patient received 2000 μg of phVEGF-165 applied to coating of angioplasty balloon. Repeat angiogram showed increased collateralization 4 weeks later [31]. Baumgarther et al. performed an open-label trial of 9 CLI patients (10 limbs) who received IM administration of 4000 μg of naked plasmid DNA encoding 165-amino-acid isoform of phVEGF-165 [32]. Study showed improved ABI (0.33 +/− 0.05 to 0.48 +/− 0.03, $p = .02$), collateralization on angiography (9/10 limbs), ulcer healing (4/7 limbs), and limb salvage with common complication being transient lower extremity edema. Later on, Simovic et al. performed an open-label dose-escalating trial in 17 CLI patients who were administered IM injections of phVEGF-165 [33]. It showed improvements in ABI ($p < 0.01$) symptom score ($p < 0.01$), sensory examination score ($p < 0.01$), total examination score ($p = 0.01$), peroneal motor amplitude ($p = .03$), and quantitative vibration threshold ($p = 0.04$). In 2003, Shyu et al. published a study of 21 CLI patients (24 limbs) injected with between 400 and 2000 μg of phVEGF-165 showing yet again improvements in ABI (0.58 ± 0.24 to 0.72 ± 0.28; $p < 0.001$), rest pain (20/24 limbs), ulcer healing (12/16 limbs), and distal circulation on angiography (19/24 limbs) [34]. Again the complication was transient edema related to VEGF expression. Makinen et al. performed the first phase-II trial in CLI patients to evaluate safety, angiographic and hemodynamic responses of local catheter-mediated VEGF therapy after percutaneous transluminal angioplasty (PTA) [35]. Patients received either ringers lactate (19 patients), adVEGF (18 patients), or VEGF plasmid. At the end of 3 months, there was increased vascularity in the VEGF-treated patients distally (adVEGF $p = 0.03$, plasmid VEGF $p = 0.02$) and specifically in the region of ischemic interest in the adVEGF group ($p = 0.01$). Another phase-II double-blind, placebo-controlled study by Kusumanto et al. performed in 54 diabetic CLI patients compared IM administration of phVEGF-165 to placebo (0.9% NaCl) [36]. Primary endpoint of amputation was similar in both groups (placebo 6, phVEGF 3, p = NS) and secondary endpoints showed hemodynamic improvement (1 vs 7; $p = 0.05$), more ulcer healing (0 vs 7; $p = 0.01$), and rest pain improvement (2 vs 5; p = NS).

VEGF was also evaluated in IC patients in a phase-I study in which 18 subjects underwent IM administration of VEGF cDNA (CI-1023) or placebo [28]. It was found to be safe; however, no significant conclusions were made of its efficacy due to small number of subjects. In the regional angiogenesis with vascular endothelial growth factor (RAVE) trial, a phase-II double-blind, placebo-controlled study of 105 IC patients administered adenoviral vascular endothelial growth factor 121 (AdVEGF121) [37]. On 12-week follow-up, study did not show improvements in PWT, ABI, claudication onset time, or quality of life measures.

Lastly, VEGF-mediated gene therapy has also known to be safe in long term as a 10-year follow-up study of 54 patients showed no differences between VEGF and placebo administered patients for causes of death, cancer development (VEGF-Adv 0/10 vs VEGF-p/l 1/8 vs Control 1/7, $p = 0.5$), diabetes (3/10 vs 3/8 vs 2/7, $p = 1.00$), or diabetic retinopathy (0/10 vs 1/8 vs 0/7, $p = 0.45$) [38].

HEPATOCYTE GROWTH FACTOR

Hepatocyte growth factor is (HGF) is a mitogenic protein that works through tyrosine phosphorylation of its specific receptor, c-Met in the endothelial and smooth muscle cells. It causes cell proliferation, angiogenesis, antiinflammation, motility, and morphogenesis [39,40]. Its unique capability to promote angiogenesis without causing inflammation has been drawing attention [40]. After success with initial animal models, Morishita et al. injected IM naked HGF plasmid DNA in six CLI patients and showed a reduction in pain by VAS in five patients as well as increase in ABI in five patients and reduction in ulcer size in four patients with no edema or adverse events at 12 weeks [40–44]. Powell et al. further investigated HGF by performing a double-blind placebo-controlled study called hepatocyte growth factor plasmid to improve limb perfusion in patients with critical limb ischemia (HGF-STAT trial) in 104 patients and found no differences in ABI, pain relief, wound healing, or major amputations [45]. So far HGF therapy seemed to appear safe; however, its efficacy was not established. A follow-up study was pursued with 27 CLI patients with no revascularization options who were randomly assigned to receive three sets of eight IM injections of either AMG001 ($n = 21$) or placebo ($n = 6$) every 2 weeks [46]. At 6 months, a significant improvement in TBI (0.05 ± 0.05 vs -0.17 ± 0.04; $p = .047$) and rest pain (VAS: -1.9 ± 1.3 vs $+0.06 \pm 0.2$; $p = .04$) from baseline was observed in the HGF group compared to placebo but there was no differences in wound healing (HGF 31% vs placebo 0%; $p = .28$), major amputations (HGF 29% vs placebo 33%), or mortality (HGF 19% vs placebo 17%). Shigematsu et al. investigated 44 CLI subjects in a multicenter, randomized, double-blind, placebo-controlled trial comparing IM administered naked plasmid encoding human HGF gene to placebo [47]. At 12 weeks, rest pain improved significantly in HGF group compared to placebo (70.4% vs 30.8%; $p = 0.014$) along with improved quality of life and no serious adverse events. In 2011, Gu et al. published an article in which two isoforms of HGF (pCK-HGF-X7) were studied in CLI. Increasing doses of pCK-HGF-X7 were received by 21 CLI subjects at day 1 and 15 [48]. At 3-month follow-up, there were no adverse events with reduction in pain via VAS ($p < 0.001$), increase in ABI ($p = 0.026$), and increase in $TcPO_2$ ($p = 0.012$). Wound healing was seen in six of nine patients. That year itself in a phase-I/IIa trial of 22 IC subjects who were administered 2 or 4 mg of HGF plasmid IM showed no serious adverse events or edema on a 6-month follow-up [49]. A 2-year follow-up showed increase in ABI (11/14 patients), reduction in rest pain (9/9 patients), and decrease in ulcer size (9/10 patients) [50]. Recently, Cui et al. randomly assigned 21 CLI subjects in to four dose groups (4−16 mg) to receive IM injection of naked plasmid DNA expressing HGF into ischemic calf and/or thigh muscles twice on days 1 and 15 in a phase-I trial [51]. Study showed no adverse effects or tolerability issues. Additionally, there was improvement in ABI and $TcPO_2$. At 3 months, pain had reduced with disappearance of pain in 14/17 subjects, 2/4 ulcers completely healed, and other two had reduced in size. Five subjects had gangrene of which one healed completely and two showed reductions in size.

Hypoxia-Induced Factor-1 Alpha

Hypoxia-induced factor-1 (HIF-1) is a transcription regulatory factor involved in cellular response to ischemia or hypoxia [52]. It controls genes encoding

VEGF, platelet-derived growth factor, endothelial nitric oxide synthase, etc. and hence controls response to hypoxia in the cells [8,53–57]. Animal studies have shown improved circulation and collaterization in hind limb ischemia model [58–61]. In 2007, Rajagopalan et al. conducted two phase-I studies; a randomized, double-blind, placebo-controlled study, and an open-label extension study of 34 CLI subjects with no revascularization options receiving HIF-1α at doses of 1 × 10(8) to 2 × 10(11) viral particles [62]. No serious adverse events were related to the study directly. At 1-year follow-up, complete resolution of rest pain was seen in 14 of 32 subjects and ulcer was healed in 5 of 18 subjects. Common side effect was edema and disease progression. Later on in 2011, Creager et al. published a double-blind trial of 289 IC subjects who were randomized to one of three doses of Ad2/HIF-1α/VP16 [2 × 10(9), 2 × 10(10), or 2 × 10(11) viral particles] or placebo, administered IM [63]. At 6 months, the primary endpoint of PWT was not different between the groups. Also secondary endpoints of claudication onset time, ABI or quality of life were not different between placebo and HIF-1α groups.

Summary of Growth Factor Therapy in PAD

Growth factor therapy has shown tremendous promise in improving circulation, collateralization, pain relief, and wound healing in animal trails and phase-I and -II human trials. It appears to be more effective in CLI subjects and has not shown much promise in PAD patients with IC. Looking at clinical outcomes before it reaches primetime clinical medicine, we can say that there is still great need for further research in this field especially in phase-III clinical trials. Further understanding of genomics will likely help us appropriately select candidates most likely to respond to these therapies. Additionally, further studies need to be pursued to identify ideal vectors of transmission, combinations of different factors, or combination of gene and cell therapies to find favorable and consistent outcomes. Lastly, majority of these trials are being considered in subjects with end-stage CLI with impending amputations and no revascularization options. It would be worthwhile studying early interventions with these therapies in combination with surgical or endovascular interventions to see if this combination would be synergistic in improving clinical outcomes as well as procedural outcomes.

REFERENCES

[1] Hirsch AT, Haskal ZJ, Hertzer NR, et al. ACC/AHA 2005 practice guidelines for the management of patients with peripheral arterial disease (lower extremity, renal, mesenteric, and abdominal aortic): a collaborative report from the American Association for Vascular Surgery/Society for Vascular Surgery, Society for Cardiovascular Angiography and Interventions, Society for Vascular Medicine and Biology, Society of Interventional Radiology, and the ACC/AHA Task Force on Practice Guidelines (Writing Committee to Develop Guidelines for the Management of Patients With Peripheral Arterial Disease): endorsed by the American

Association of Cardiovascular and Pulmonary Rehabilitation; National Heart, Lung, and Blood Institute; Society for Vascular Nursing; TransAtlantic Inter-Society Consensus; and Vascular Disease Foundation. Circulation 2006;113(11):e463–654.

[2] Diehm C, Allenberg JR, Pittrow D, et al. Mortality and vascular morbidity in older adults with asymptomatic versus symptomatic peripheral artery disease. Circulation 2009;120(21):2053–61.

[3] Libby P, Ridker PM, Hansson GK. Progress and challenges in translating the biology of atherosclerosis. Nature 2011;473(7347):317–25.

[4] Folkman J. Angiogenesis in cancer, vascular, rheumatoid and other disease. Nat Med 1995;1(1):27–31.

[5] Schaper W, Buschmann I. Arteriogenesis, the good and bad of it. Cardiovasc Res 1999;43(4):835–7.

[6] Chalothorn D, Clayton JA, Zhang H, Pomp D, Faber JE. Collateral density, remodeling, and VEGF-A expression differ widely between mouse strains. Physiol Genomics 2007;30(2):179–91.

[7] Folkman J. Tumor angiogenesis: therapeutic implications. N Engl J Med 1971;285(21):1182–6.

[8] Wang GL, Jiang BH, Rue EA, Semenza GL. Hypoxia-inducible factor 1 is a basic-helix-loop-helix-PAS heterodimer regulated by cellular O_2 tension. Proc Natl Acad Sci USA 1995;92(12):5510–4.

[9] Shimamura M, Nakagami H, Taniyama Y, Morishita R. Gene therapy for peripheral arterial disease. Expert Opin Biol Ther 2014;14(8):1175–84.

[10] Shimamura M, Nakagami H, Koriyama H, Morishita R. Gene therapy and cell-based therapies for therapeutic angiogenesis in peripheral artery disease. Biomed Res Int 2013;2013:186215.

[11] Presta M, Dell'Era P, Mitola S, Moroni E, Ronca R, Rusnati M. Fibroblast growth factor/fibroblast growth factor receptor system in angiogenesis. Cytokine Growth Factor Rev 2005;16(2):159–78.

[12] Aviles RJ, Annex BH, Lederman RJ. Testing clinical therapeutic angiogenesis using basic fibroblast growth factor (FGF-2). Br J Pharmacol 2003;140(4):637–46.

[13] Cao R, Brakenhielm E, Pawliuk R, et al. Angiogenic synergism, vascular stability and improvement of hind-limb ischemia by a combination of PDGF-BB and FGF-2. Nat Med 2003;9(5):604–13.

[14] Grines CL, Watkins MW, Helmer G, et al. Angiogenic Gene Therapy (AGENT) trial in patients with stable angina pectoris. Circulation 2002;105(11):1291–7.

[15] Lazarous DF, Unger EF, Epstein SE, et al. Basic fibroblast growth factor in patients with intermittent claudication: results of a phase I trial. J Am Coll Cardiol 2000;36(4):1239–44.

[16] Lederman RJ, Mendelsohn FO, Anderson RD, et al. Therapeutic angiogenesis with recombinant fibroblast growth factor-2 for intermittent claudication (the TRAFFIC study): a randomised trial. Lancet 2002;359(9323):2053–8.

[17] Comerota AJ, Throm RC, Miller KA, et al. Naked plasmid DNA encoding fibroblast growth factor type 1 for the treatment of end-stage unreconstructible lower extremity ischemia: preliminary results of a phase I trial. J Vasc Surg 2002;35(5):930–6.

[18] Marui A, Tabata Y, Kojima S, et al. A novel approach to therapeutic angiogenesis for patients with critical limb ischemia by sustained release of basic fibroblast growth factor using biodegradable gelatin hydrogel: an initial report of the phase I-IIa study. Circ J 2007;71(8):1181–6.

[19] Nikol S, Baumgartner I, Van Belle E, et al. Therapeutic angiogenesis with intramuscular NV1FGF improves amputation-free survival in patients with critical limb ischemia. Mol Ther 2008;16(5):972–8.

[20] Hashimoto T, Koyama H, Miyata T, et al. Selective and sustained delivery of basic fibroblast growth factor (bFGF) for treatment of peripheral arterial disease: results of a phase I trial. Eur J Vasc Endovasc Surg 2009;38(1):71–5.
[21] Belch J, Hiatt WR, Baumgartner I, et al. Effect of fibroblast growth factor NV1FGF on amputation and death: a randomised placebo-controlled trial of gene therapy in critical limb ischaemia. Lancet 2011;377(9781):1929–37.
[22] Takagi G, Miyamoto M, Tara S, et al. Controlled-release basic fibroblast growth factor for peripheral artery disease: comparison with autologous bone marrow-derived stem cell transfer. Tissue Eng Part A 2011;17(21–22):2787–94.
[23] Kumagai M, Marui A, Tabata Y, et al. Safety and efficacy of sustained release of basic fibroblast growth factor using gelatin hydrogel in patients with critical limb ischemia. Heart Vessels 2015;25861983.
[24] Dokun AO, Annex BH. The VEGF165b "ICE-o-form" puts a chill on the VEGF story. Circ Res 2011;109(3):246–7.
[25] Ferrara N, Davis-Smyth T. The biology of vascular endothelial growth factor. Endocr Rev 1997;18(1):4–25.
[26] Holmes K, Roberts OL, Thomas AM, Cross MJ. Vascular endothelial growth factor receptor-2: structure, function, intracellular signalling and therapeutic inhibition. Cell Signal 2007;19(10):2003–12.
[27] Ferrara N, Keyt B. Vascular endothelial growth factor: basic biology and clinical implications. EXS 1997;79:209–32.
[28] Mohler ER 3rd, Rajagopalan S, Olin JW, et al. Adenoviral-mediated gene transfer of vascular endothelial growth factor in critical limb ischemia: safety results from a phase I trial. Vasc Med 2003;8(1):9–13.
[29] Hopkins SP, Bulgrin JP, Sims RL, Bowman B, Donovan DL, Schmidt SP. Controlled delivery of vascular endothelial growth factor promotes neovascularization and maintains limb function in a rabbit model of ischemia. J Vasc Surg 1998;27(5):886–94. discussion 895.
[30] Li Y, Hazarika S, Xie D, Pippen AM, Kontos CD, Annex BH. In mice with type 2 diabetes, a vascular endothelial growth factor (VEGF)-activating transcription factor modulates VEGF signaling and induces therapeutic angiogenesis after hindlimb ischemia. Diabetes 2007;56(3):656–65.
[31] Isner JM, Pieczek A, Schainfeld R, et al. Clinical evidence of angiogenesis after arterial gene transfer of phVEGF165 in patient with ischaemic limb. Lancet 1996;348(9024):370–4.
[32] Baumgartner I, Pieczek A, Manor O, et al. Constitutive expression of phVEGF165 after intramuscular gene transfer promotes collateral vessel development in patients with critical limb ischemia. Circulation 1998;97(12):1114–23.
[33] Simovic D, Isner JM, Ropper AH, Pieczek A, Weinberg DH. Improvement in chronic ischemic neuropathy after intramuscular phVEGF165 gene transfer in patients with critical limb ischemia. Arch Neurol 2001;58(5):761–8.
[34] Shyu KG, Chang H, Wang BW, Kuan P. Intramuscular vascular endothelial growth factor gene therapy in patients with chronic critical leg ischemia. Am J Med 2003;114(2):85–92.
[35] Makinen K, Manninen H, Hedman M, et al. Increased vascularity detected by digital subtraction angiography after VEGF gene transfer to human lower limb artery: a randomized, placebo-controlled, double-blinded phase II study. Mol Ther 2002;6(1):127–33.
[36] Kusumanto YH, van Weel V, Mulder NH, et al. Treatment with intramuscular vascular endothelial growth factor gene compared with placebo for patients with diabetes mellitus and critical limb ischemia: a double-blind randomized trial. Hum Gene Ther 2006;17(6):683–91.

[37] Rajagopalan S, Mohler ER 3rd, Lederman RJ, et al. Regional angiogenesis with vascular endothelial growth factor in peripheral arterial disease: a phase II randomized, double-blind, controlled study of adenoviral delivery of vascular endothelial growth factor 121 in patients with disabling intermittent claudication. Circulation 2003;108(16):1933–8.
[38] Muona K, Makinen K, Hedman M, Manninen H, Yla-Herttuala S. 10-year safety follow-up in patients with local VEGF gene transfer to ischemic lower limb. Gene Ther 2012;19(4):392–5.
[39] Nakamura T, Mizuno S. The discovery of hepatocyte growth factor (HGF) and its significance for cell biology, life sciences and clinical medicine. Proc Jpn Acad Ser B Phys Biol Sci 2010;86(6):588–610.
[40] Kaga T, Kawano H, Sakaguchi M, Nakazawa T, Taniyama Y, Morishita R. Hepatocyte growth factor stimulated angiogenesis without inflammation: differential actions between hepatocyte growth factor, vascular endothelial growth factor and basic fibroblast growth factor. Vascul Pharmacol 2012;57(1):3–9.
[41] Hayashi S, Morishita R, Nakamura S, et al. Potential role of hepatocyte growth factor, a novel angiogenic growth factor, in peripheral arterial disease: downregulation of HGF in response to hypoxia in vascular cells. Circulation 1999;100(19 Suppl):II301–8.
[42] Taniyama Y, Morishita R, Hiraoka K, et al. Therapeutic angiogenesis induced by human hepatocyte growth factor gene in rat diabetic hind limb ischemia model: molecular mechanisms of delayed angiogenesis in diabetes. Circulation 2001;104(19):2344–50.
[43] Taniyama Y, Morishita R, Aoki M, et al. Therapeutic angiogenesis induced by human hepatocyte growth factor gene in rat and rabbit hindlimb ischemia models: preclinical study for treatment of peripheral arterial disease. Gene Ther 2001;8(3):181–9.
[44] Morishita R, Aoki M, Hashiya N, et al. Safety evaluation of clinical gene therapy using hepatocyte growth factor to treat peripheral arterial disease. Hypertension 2004;44(2):203–9.
[45] Powell RJ, Simons M, Mendelsohn FO, et al. Results of a double-blind, placebo-controlled study to assess the safety of intramuscular injection of hepatocyte growth factor plasmid to improve limb perfusion in patients with critical limb ischemia. Circulation 2008;118(1):58–65.
[46] Powell RJ, Goodney P, Mendelsohn FO, Moen EK, Annex BH. Safety and efficacy of patient specific intramuscular injection of HGF plasmid gene therapy on limb perfusion and wound healing in patients with ischemic lower extremity ulceration: results of the HGF-0205 trial. J Vasc Surg 2010;52(6):1525–30.
[47] Shigematsu H, Yasuda K, Iwai T, et al. Randomized, double-blind, placebo-controlled clinical trial of hepatocyte growth factor plasmid for critical limb ischemia. Gene Ther 2010;17(9):1152–61.
[48] Gu Y, Zhang J, Guo L, et al. A phase I clinical study of naked DNA expressing two isoforms of hepatocyte growth factor to treat patients with critical limb ischemia. J Gene Med 2011;13(11):602–10.
[49] Morishita R, Makino H, Aoki M, et al. Phase I/IIa clinical trial of therapeutic angiogenesis using hepatocyte growth factor gene transfer to treat critical limb ischemia. Arterioscler Thromb Vasc Biol 2011;31(3):713–20.
[50] Makino H, Aoki M, Hashiya N, et al. Long-term follow-up evaluation of results from clinical trial using hepatocyte growth factor gene to treat severe peripheral arterial disease. Arterioscler Thromb Vasc Biol 2012;32(10):2503–9.
[51] Cui S, Guo L, Li X, et al. Clinical Safety and Preliminary Efficacy of Plasmid pUDK-HGF Expressing Human Hepatocyte Growth Factor (HGF) in Patients with Critical Limb Ischemia. Eur J Vasc Endovasc Surg 2015;50(4):494–501.
[52] Semenza GL. Life with oxygen. Science 2007;318(5847):62–4.

[53] Wenger RH, Gassmann M. Oxygen(es) and the hypoxia-inducible factor-1. Biol Chem 1997;378(7):609–16.
[54] Rey S, Lee K, Wang CJ, et al. Synergistic effect of HIF-1alpha gene therapy and HIF-1-activated bone marrow-derived angiogenic cells in a mouse model of limb ischemia. Proc Natl Acad Sci USA 2009;106(48):20399–404.
[55] Lando D, Peet DJ, Whelan DA, Gorman JJ, Whitelaw ML. Asparagine hydroxylation of the HIF transactivation domain a hypoxic switch. Science 2002;295(5556):858–61.
[56] Guillemin K, Krasnow MA. The hypoxic response: huffing and HIFing. Cell 1997;89(1):9–12.
[57] Chang EI, Loh SA, Ceradini DJ, et al. Age decreases endothelial progenitor cell recruitment through decreases in hypoxia-inducible factor 1alpha stabilization during ischemia. Circulation 2007;116(24):2818–29.
[58] Vincent KA, Shyu KG, Luo Y, et al. Angiogenesis is induced in a rabbit model of hindlimb ischemia by naked DNA encoding an HIF-1alpha/VP16 hybrid transcription factor. Circulation 2000;102(18):2255–61.
[59] Li M, Liu C, Bin J, et al. Mutant hypoxia inducible factor-1alpha improves angiogenesis and tissue perfusion in ischemic rabbit skeletal muscle. Microvasc Res 2011;81(1):26–33.
[60] Kajiwara H, Luo Z, Belanger AJ, et al. A hypoxic inducible factor-1 alpha hybrid enhances collateral development and reduces vascular leakage in diabetic rats. J Gene Med 2009;11(5):390–400.
[61] Ouma GO, Rodriguez E, Muthumani K, Weiner DB, Wilensky RL, Mohler ER 3rd. In vivo electroporation of constitutively expressed HIF-1alpha plasmid DNA improves neovascularization in a mouse model of limb ischemia. J Vasc Surg 2014;59(3):786–93.
[62] Rajagopalan S, Olin J, Deitcher S, et al. Use of a constitutively active hypoxia-inducible factor-1alpha transgene as a therapeutic strategy in no-option critical limb ischemia patients: phase I dose-escalation experience. Circulation 2007;115(10):1234–43.
[63] Creager MA, Olin JW, Belch JJ, et al. Effect of hypoxia-inducible factor-1alpha gene therapy on walking performance in patients with intermittent claudication. Circulation 2011;124(16):1765–73.

Chapter 2

Regenerative Cell Therapy: Historical Background and Future Directions

K.S. Telukuntla, MD, E.R. Mohler III, MD
Perelman School of Medicine at the University of Pennsylvania, Division of Cardiovascular Medicine, Department of Medicine, Philadelphia, PA, United States

INTRODUCTION

Since the term "Stammzellen" (stem cell) was first coined back in the late 19th century by Ernst Haeckel, the scientific community has made significant and continued progress in its understanding and application of stem cells [1]. Yet, even after 100 years and many advances, this field is still considered to be in its infancy as fundamentals of stem-cell biology still need to be understood. The promise and potential of stem cells has given birth to the field of regenerative medicine which offers the possibility to reverse tissue damage and sequela without transplant. In cardiovascular medicine, stem-cell research has mainly been focused on myocyte regeneration in patients with advanced heart failure. Equally important and promising research is taking place for peripheral artery disease (PAD). Until now, the treatment options for patients with severe PAD are limited to interventional or surgical revascularization to increase blood flow. Continued advances in the field of cell therapy will allow physicians to offer new therapeutic options to reverse the limb ischemia and claudication. This chapter will highlight the origins and evolution of cell therapy in the context of peripheral artery disease.

HISTORICAL OVERVIEW

In 1867, the German pathologist, Julius Cohnheim postulated, "All cells come from the bloodstream and therefore … from the Bone Marrow" [2,3]. While Cohnheim was highly regarded for his work on inflammation, no one could appreciate the far-reaching consequences of this idea. Essentially, he had identified the bone marrow as the organ with regenerative capacity with its reservoir of stem cells. According to this theory, these stem cells should have the ability to differentiate into an organ-specific cell type. This was the presumptive model

Regenerative Medicine for Peripheral Artery Disease. http://dx.doi.org/10.1016/B978-0-12-801344-1.00002-4

for organ homeostasis and the body's regenerative capacity until the discovery and identification of the endothelial progenitor cells (EPCs) by Asahara et al. [4]. In this groundbreaking study, Asahara and coworkers showed that CD34+ and VEFGR2+ mononuclear cells were able to differentiate into mature endothelial cells in vitro. In addition, both cell lines led to the formation of new small vessels in the ischemic-hind-limb models.

EPCs can be broadly defined as any cell that has the ability to differentiate into an endothelial cell [2,5,6]. According to Asahara's theory, EPCs are an instrumental component of arterial wall repair. As the body ages and the repair potential of the bone marrow and EPCs declines, it permits an uninterrupted cycle of injury and inflammation ultimately leading to atherosclerosis [2].

EPCs have been isolated from multiple sources including bone marrow, adipose tissue, peripheral blood, and cord blood, but no single source has proven to be more superior [5–7]. In addition, there is a sizeable level of overlap of cell surface markers among EPCs and hematopoietic cells [2,5]. As a consequence, the identification and isolation of a pure EPC population remains challenging as the unique phenotypic determinants are unidentified. Asahara's discovery demonstrated that angiogenesis is possible even in the postnatal environment, but further investigation is needed to translate this discovery into a novel therapeutic intervention.

In addition to the hypothesis and theories emerging in the late 19th and 20th centuries, there were several other discoveries that allowed the utilization of stem cells as a treatment modality for PAD. In 1984, Dr Curt Civin and his team discovered the cell surface glycoprotein CD34 which has now become a marker for hematopoietic stem-progenitor cells (HSPC). They ultimately discovered My10 (My10 = CD34) which binds to approximately 1% of the human bone marrow cells. Additional investigation revealed that all HSPCs and endothelial cells are CD34+, but other differentiated cell types are CD34−. In the following years, CD34 was used to illustrate the development of lymphocytes [8]. The CD34+ cells that were isolated by Asahara and his coworkers are shown to differentiate into endothelial cells [4].

In order to apply all of the aforementioned advances to develop cell therapy for PAD, the hind-limb ischemia model was established for preclinical mouse, rat, and porcine models. The most widely accepted animal model produces acute ischemia by ligation of the common femoral artery. Though the preclinical experiments showed enough promise to proceed to clinical trials, this is not representative of the chronic ischemia and sequela that is detected in PAD [2,9,10].There is a strong desire to identify a more appropriate animal model that is able to replicate human atherosclerotic pathophysiology. The underlying pathophysiology impacts the treatment modality and this is best seen in the trial conducted by Idei et al. which demonstrated the sustained long-term benefit in the patients with thromboangitis obliterans (TAO, previously known as Buerger's disease) as compared to patients with PAD. Both groups received BM-MNCs, but the 4-year survival rate was 100% in TAO compared to the

76% in PAD [11]. This highlights the need to design an animal model with pathophysiology similar to human PAD in order to promote a more elegant approach targeting the underlying atherosclerotic disease process. In addition, it would help promote more parallel and reproducible findings between animal and clinical studies.

CURRENT TREATMENTS FOR PAD

For over 10 million Americans and many more in the world with PAD, there are limited options for treatment [12]. Before the concept of stem-cell therapy was identified as a possible option, patients with severe PAD or critical limb ischemia (CLI) had limited nonrevascularization interventions. First-line treatment for atherosclerotic PAD is focused on risk factor and lifestyle modification including, but not limited to, exercise, smoking cessation, glycemic control, and blood-pressure control [9,13,14]. Medical therapy with antiplatelet agents such as aspirin, clopidogrel, or cilastazol offers some benefit. In cases of severe PAD or CLI, the treatment of choice is surgical or endovascular revascularization with the goal of increasing blood flow to the affected limb. Unfortunately, nearly a quarter of these patients are not suitable candidates for revascularization and they ultimately require amputation. This translates to over 100,000 annual amputations in the United States alone [12]. Furthermore, the acute mortality associated with limb amputation is estimated as high as 30% with a 5-year survival rate slightly under 30% [13]. As if the statistics and mortality associated with PAD are not already alarming, there is increasing evidence about the impact on quality of life of dealing with PAD. Although quality of life and psychological impact of dealing with cancer or advanced heart failure is often discussed, some studies have shown that PAD can have the same impact to quality of life as a terminally ill cancer patient [5]. Cell therapy offers a potential answer for this unmet need in PAD with the goal to reverse tissue damage and improve limb perfusion.

PRECLINICAL AND CLINICAL TRIALS FOR PAD

Although the following chapters will discuss the preclinical and clinical trials in further detail, this section will provide a general overview of the progress made in stem-cell therapies for PAD. The initial animal studies in rat, mouse, and rabbit models utilized the hind-limb ischemia protocol to demonstrate the angiogenesis and neovascularization that prompted clinical trials. A more comprehensive list of animal trials can be referenced from Lawall et al. [13].

As mentioned previously, CD34+ stem-cells isolated from the blood have been shown to induce angiogenesis in the ground-breaking experiments by Asahara et al. [4]. Labeled human cells were injected into the tail vein of athymic mice and via histological analysis confirmed the migration of these cells to the perivascular location in the ischemic limb. Subsequent animal studies also demonstrate that cell therapy is able to improve blood flow to the affected limb and increase collateral vessel formation [10]. The encouraging results from the preclinical experiments conducted by Asahara and others ultimately set the stage to move forward with clinical trials.

The majority of the clinical trials have used peripheral or bone-marrow-derived mononuclear cells (BM-MNCs). The first landmark randomized control trial to establish safety and efficacy of the BM-MNCs was the Therapeutic Angiogenesis using Cell Transplantation (TACT) study performed by Tateishi-Yuyama et. al in 2002 (Table 2.1) [15]. The TACT investigators first did a pilot study with 25 patients that had unilateral ischemia of the lowers extremities. They subsequently conducted a randomized control portion with 22 patients with bilateral leg ischemia. In the study, the intramuscular injection of undifferentiated BM-MNCs, when compared to unstimulated peripheral blood mononuclear cells (PB-MNCs), resulted in statistically significant improvements in ankle brachial pressure index (ABPI), transcutaneous oxygen pressure, pain-free walking distance that remained at 2-year follow-up [5,6,15,16]. The fact that BM-MNCs showed more improvement over unstimulated PB-MNCs suggests that there is an optimal quantity and concentration of stem cells that are required to promote angiogenesis. Most importantly, TACT established the safety profile for BM-MNCs in PAD. No adverse events were reported, but two patients died of a myocardial infarction that was determined by autopsy to be unrelated to the intervention.

Following the completion of TACT, there have been a number of additional trials with modifications to the trial design trying to reproduce the safety and efficacy. Most of the trials have employed BM-MNCs or PB-MNCs, but a vigorous and unresolved debate remains about the optimal delivery, dosing, and duration of treatment. Unfortunately, a large majority of these trials do not have enough power and/or are uncontrolled as evidenced by the number of patients enrolled in each of the trials listed in Table 2.1. Although these continue to remain the major obstacles, each of these trials has made a small but important contribution in the journey to realizing the full potential of cell-based therapies.

FUTURE DIRECTION IN PAD

Similar to many fields in medicine trying to utilize stem cells, there are still a lot of unanswered questions. However, the promising data emerging from preclinical and clinical trials in PAD continues to generate more interest, momentum, and progress. Since TACT, there have been several dozen clinical trials that aim to demonstrate efficacy of this novel therapy, but only a few have been designed as randomized control trials. In order to advance cell therapy in PAD to phase-III trials, researchers need to design adequately powered randomized control trials with larger patient populations, conduct optimization studies to identify ideal dosing and delivery strategies, and establish novel assessment tools.

TABLE 2.1 Clinical Trials Employing Stem Cell Therapy for Peripheral Artery Disease (PAD)

Cell type	Authors/trial name*	Total # of patients	Description	Delivery method	Outcomes
BM-MNC and PB-MNC	Tateishi-Yuyama et al. [15] TACT: Therapeutic angiogenesis using cell transplantation	22	Patients with bilateral leg ischemia with delivery of BMMNCs or PBMNCs in each leg with 24 month follow-up	IM	BM-MNC showed significant improvement of ABIs, $TcPO_2$, rest pain, pain-free walking time compared to placebo and PB-MNC arms
BM-MNC	Gu et al. [24]	32	Two groups of patients received BM-MNCs. Group 1 via IM delivery and group 2 via IA delivery. No placebo arm in trial	IM and IA	IM and IA groups both showed similar results: improved rest pain, TcO2 and ABI
BM-MNC	Franz et al. [25]	9	As an alternative to amputation, patients with severe PAD received BMMNC via both IM and IA routes	IM and IA	Three patients avoided amputation with complete resolution of ulcers, 8/9 patients showed some degree of improvement per study criteria
BM-MNC	Higashi et al. [26]	7	BM-MNC implantation with ACh-mediated endothelium-dependent vasodilatation compared to placebo in PAD.	IM	Improved ABPI, TcO2, pain-free walking time
BM-MNC	Idei et al. [11]	97 (55 with PAD, 42 with TAO)	Patients with PAD or TAO divided into BM-MNC and placebo group to evaluate long-term outcomes	IM	After BM-MNCs, 4-year survival rate was 100% in TAO and 76% in PAD arm. Findings were sustained in patients with TAO, but not sustained in PAD
PB-MNC	Huang et al. [20]	28	CLI patients randomized to control and G-CSF stimulated PBMNC group with 3-month follow-up	Multiple IM injections	Significant improvements in ABI, limb salvage and ulcer healing

(*Continued*)

TABLE 2.1 Clinical Trials Employing Stem Cell Therapy for Peripheral Artery Disease (PAD) (*cont.*)

Cell type	Authors/trial name*	Total # of patients	Description	Delivery method	Outcomes
G-CSF mobilized PB-MNC	Ozturk et al. [21]	40	DM patients with CLI randomized to placebo and treatment arms receiving G-CSF mobilized PB-BNCs with 12-week follow-up	Multiple IM injections	Significant improvements in ABPI, $TcPO_2$, and pain-free walking score, but no significant change in amputation rates
PB-MNC	Losordo et al. [27]	28	RCT, double-blinded IM delivery of CD34+ PB-MNCs stratified by high and low dosing concentrations	IM	Dose-dependent association with decreased amputation sustained at 12-month follow up, but statistically nonsignificant
BM-MSC	Gupta et al. [28]	20	Double blinded RCT with placebo versus BM-MSCs(2 million cells/kg) delivered to CLI patients	IM	No significant change for treatment-related adverse events (primary end point), but significantly improved ABPIs
TRC	Powell et al. [29] RESTORE-CLI	72	Phase II RCT for CLI patients receiving IM delivery of TRCs in treatment arm	IM	Decrease in major amputation, all-cause mortality, de novo gangrene, but not statically significant
PB-BMC	Teraa et al. [22] JUVENTAS: reJUVenating ENdothelial progenitor cells via transcutaneous intraarterial supplementation	160	Randomized, placebo-controlled, double-blinded trial with repeated intraarterial BM-MNCs injections (three times a week for 3 weeks)	Repetitive IA injections	No significant difference in major amputation rate or mortality at 6 months

ABPI, ankle brachial pressure index; *AcH*, acetylcholine; *IM*, intramuscular; *IA*, intraarterial; *PAD*, peripheral artery disease; *RCT*, randomized control trial; *TAO*, thromoangitis obliterans; TcO_2, transcutaneous oxygen pressure.
**Trial names provided only if applicable.*

The initial hypothesis behind the delivery of stem cells was that once they were delivered into the ischemic areas they would differentiate into mature cells. However, the low engraftment rates seen in many of the studies could not explain the resulting functional benefits and have raised questions of the true mechanism of action behind the regenerative effects seen in the preclinical and clinical trials. There is a growing body of evidence that the true mechanisms responsible for the regenerative effect are largely due to the indirect or paracrine-mediated effects. The exact etiology of the paracrine effect is still under investigation, but recent discoveries have implicated extracellular vesicles (EVs) which are derived from the membranes of cells though an exocytic budding process [17]. In the last two decades, extracellular vesicles have emerged as a likely source of intercellular signaling and communication, cell-senescence, and maturation of cells via transmission of biochemical substrates. Certain EVs released from stem cells have regenerative potential and also protect from injury whereas other EVs from CD34+ cells promote angiogenesis [18,19]. The field of medicine has yet to fully comprehend the true potential of EVs, but research is going on to utilize EVs to develop novel therapeutic targets or employ them as drug-delivery mechanisms.

In regards to optimization studies, there is still some degree of debate on the best delivery method. The intramuscular approach injects cells directly into the ischemic areas that require angiogenesis, but engraftment rates are documented to be as low as 0.44–10% after 96 h [13]. The intraarterial approach is thought to direct cells to border zones that still have an adequate oxygen and nutrient supply to support an enriching environment for new cell activity. Clinical trials have largely preferred the intramuscular approach over the intraarterial approach, but no randomized clinical trial has ever compared both approaches. Some researchers including Huang et al., Ozturk et al., and Teraa et al. have also experimented with the concept of repeated injections of stem cells [20–22].

Notably, cell therapy takes a much different mechanistic approach than current pharmacological or mechanical interventions. When a new therapy is established, it is equally important to establish valid endpoints and design new modalities to appropriately measure efficacy of interventions. In PAD, there is still no accurate or precise way to measure blood flow at the tissue level in CLI. In addition, newer imaging modalities that may be able to trace and track EPC engraftment can augment angiographic data to develop important new endpoints [6]. Evaluation of efficacy is not a challenge that is unique for PAD research. For example, research focusing on cell-based therapies in ischemic heart disease continues to struggle to properly identify a surrogate end point. Most of the landmark trials in heart failure for pharmacological interventions have used ejection fraction (EF) as the primary end point. However, emerging evidence is showing that EF may not be such a reliable way to assess efficacy of cell-based efficacy [23].

Additionally, clinical trials to date in PAD have only tried cell-based therapies for end-stage disease as a form of salvage therapy when no other routinely accepted treatment will be of benefit [16]. Greater efficacy of this novel therapy is potentially missed as the vasculature may lose some or all of its regenerative capabilities after sustaining a certain amount of damage. This approach may encourage future clinical trials to use cell therapy for mild to moderate PAD. Additional information about ongoing and future clinical trials can be found on clinicaltrials.gov.

CONCLUSIONS

While the idea of a stem cell was coined over 100 years ago, majority of the progress in cell-based therapy in PAD has been in the last two decades especially after the discovery of EPCs by Asahara. It is an area that continues to be marred with skeptism by some, but increasingly seen by many as a promising modality to reverse end-stage damage. The current body of evidence has established the safety of this novel therapy and results from clinical trials such as TACT show signs of promise and efficacy. To further define a role for cell therapy in PAD, researchers not only need to design robust randomized control trials with larger populations but also aggressively seek mechanistic insight into the fundamental biology of cell therapy. The following chapters will provide an update on the latest advances on regenerative medicine in the quest to create a novel cellular therapeutic intervention for PAD.

REFERENCES

[1] Maehle A. Ambiguous cells: the emergence of the stem cell concept in the nineteenth and twentieth centuries. Notes Rec Roy Soc 2011;65(4):359–78.

[2] Dong C, Crawford LE, Goldschmidt-Clermont PJ. Endothelial progenitor obsolescence and atherosclerotic inflammation*. J Am Coll Cardiol 2005;45(9):1458–60.

[3] Anversa P, Kajstura J, Leri A. Circulating progenitor cells: search for an identity. Circulation 2004;110(20):3158–60.

[4] Asahara T, Murohara T, Sullivan A, Silver M, van der Zee R, Li T, et al. Isolation of putative progenitor endothelial cells for angiogenesis. Science 1997;275(5302):964–6.

[5] Raval Z, Losordo DW. Cell therapy of peripheral arterial disease: from experimental findings to clinical trials. Circ Res 2013;112(9):1288–302.

[6] Gupta N, Armstrong E, Parikh S. The current state of stem cell therapy for peripheral artery disease. Curr Cardiol Rep 2014;16:1–9.

[7] Murohara T. Autologous adipose tissue as a new source of progenitor cells for therapeutic angiogenesis. J Cardiol 2009;53(2):155–63.

[8] Civin CI. CD34 stem cell stories and lessons from the CD34 wars: the Landsteiner Lecture 2009. Transfusion 2010;50(9):2046–56.

[9] Mohler ER III. Peripheral arterial disease: Identification and implications. Arch Intern Med 2003;163(19):2306–14.

[10] Gulati R, Simari RD. Defining the potential for cell therapy for vascular disease using animal models. Dis Model Mech 2009;2(3–4):130–7.

[11] Idei N, Soga J, Hata T, Fujii Y, Fujimura N, Mikami S, et al. Autologous bone-marrow mononuclear cell implantation reduces long-term major amputation risk in patients with critical limb ischemia: a comparison of atherosclerotic peripheral arterial disease and Buerger disease. Circulation 2011;4(1):15–25.

[12] Go AS, Mozaffarian D, Roger VL, Benjamin EJ, Berry JD, Blaha MJ, et al. Heart disease and stroke statistics—2014 update: a report from the American Heart Association. Circulation 2014;129(3):e28–e292.

[13] Lawall H, Bramlage P, Amann B. Stem cell and progenitor cell therapy in peripheral artery disease. Thromb Haemost 2010;4:696.

[14] Malgor RD, Alalahdab F, Elraiyah TA, Rizvi AZ, Lane MA, Prokop LJ, et al. A systematic review of treatment of intermittent claudication in the lower extremities. J Vasc Surg 2015;61(3 Supplement):54S–73S.

[15] Tateishi-Yuyama E, Matsubara H, Murohara T, Ikeda U, Shintani S, Masaki H, et al. Therapeutic angiogenesis for patients with limb ischaemia by autologous transplantation of bone-marrow cells: a pilot study and a randomised controlled trial. Lancet 2002; 360(9331):427–35.

[16] Botham CM, Bennett WL, Cooke JP. Clinical trials of adult stem cell therapy for peripheral artery disease. Methodist DeBakey Cardiovas J 2013;9(4):201–5.

[17] Curtis AM, Edelberg J, Jonas R, Rogers WT, Moore JS, Syed W, et al. Endothelial microparticles: sophisticated vesicles modulating vascular function. Vasc Med 2013;18(4):204–14.

[18] EL Andaloussi S, Mäger I, Breakefield XO, Wood MJ. Extracellular vesicles: biology and emerging therapeutic opportunities. Nat Rev Drug Disc 2013;12(5):347–57.

[19] Hodgkinson CP, Bareja A, Gomez JA, Dzau VJ. Emerging concepts in paracrine mechanisms in regenerative cardiovascular medicine and biology. Circ Res 2016;118(1):95–107.

[20] Huang P, Li S, Han M, Xiao Z, Yang R, Han ZC. Autologous transplantation of granulocyte colony–stimulating factor–mobilized peripheral blood mononuclear cells improves critical limb ischemia in diabetes. Diabetes Care 2005;28(9):2155–60.

[21] Ozturk A, Kucukardali Y, Tangi F, Erikci A, Uzun G, Bashekim C, et al. Therapeutical potential of autologous peripheral blood mononuclear cell transplantation in patients with type 2 diabetic critical limb ischemia. J Diabetes Complications 2012;26(1):29–33.

[22] Teraa M, Sprengers RW, Schutgens REG, Slaper-Cortenbach ICM, van der Graaf Y, Algra A, et al. Effect of repetitive intra-arterial infusion of bone marrow mononuclear cells in patients with no-option limb ischemia: the randomized, double-blind, placebo-controlled rejuvenating endothelial progenitor cells via transcutaneous intra-arterial supplementation (JUVENTAS) trial. Circulation 2015;131(10):851–60.

[23] Telukuntla KS, Suncion VY, Schulman IH, Hare JM. The advancing field of cell-based therapy: insights and lessons from clinical trials. J Am Heart Assoc 2013;2(5).

[24] Gu Y, Zhang J, Guo L, Qi L, Zhang S, Xu J, et al. Transplantation of autologous bone marrow mononuclear cells for patients with lower limb ischemia. Chin Med J 2008;121(11):963–7.

[25] Franz RW, Parks A, Shah KJ, Hankins T, Hartman JF, Wright ML. Use of autologous bone marrow mononuclear cell implantation therapy as a limb salvage procedure in patients with severe peripheral arterial disease. J Vasc Surg 2009;50(6):1378–90.

[26] Higashi Y, Kimura M, Hara K, Noma K, Jitsuiki D, Nakagawa K, et al. Autologous bone-marrow mononuclear cell implantation improves endothelium-dependent vasodilation in patients with limb ischemia. Circulation 2004;109(10):1215–8.

[27] Losordo DW, Kibbe MR, Mendelsohn F, Marston W, Driver VR, Sharafuddin M, et al. A randomized, controlled pilot study of autologous CD34+ cell therapy for critical limb ischemia. Circulation 2012;5(6):821–30.

[28] Gupta P, Chullikana A, Parakh R, Desai S, Das A, Gottipamula S, et al. A double blind randomized placebo controlled phase I/II study assessing the safety and efficacy of allogeneic bone marrow derived mesenchymal stem cell in critical limb ischemia. J Transl Med 2013;11(1):143.

[29] Powell RJ, Marston WA, Berceli SA, Guzman R, Henry TD, Longcore AT, Stern TP, Watling S, Bartel RL. Cellular therapy with ixmyelocel-T to treat critical limb ischemia: the randomized, double-blind, placebo-controlled RESTORE-CLI trial. Mol Ther 2012;20(6):1280–6.

Chapter 3

Bone Marrow–Derived Cells: From the Laboratory to the Clinic

J. Xie, MD, PhD*,**,§, K.L. March, MD, PhD*,**,‡, M.P. Murphy, MD*,**,†,§
*Indiana Center for Vascular Biology and Medicine (ICVBM), Indianapolis, IN, United States; **Department of Medicine, Richard L. Roudebush VA Center for Regenerative Medicine, Indianapolis, IN, United States; †Department of Surgery, Indiana University Center for Aortic Disease (IU-CAD), Indianapolis, IN, United States; ‡Krannert Institute of Cardiology, Indianapolis, IN, United States; §Indiana University Department of Surgery (IUSM), Indianapolis, IN, United States

ISOLATION AND CHARACTERIZATION OF BONE MARROW MONONUCLEAR CELLS

Definition and Composition of BMMNC

The mononuclear cell fraction of adult bone marrow (BMMNC) is defined as cells with unilobed or round nuclei and without granules in the cytoplasm. BMMNC are a heterogeneous cell population that includes hematopoietic stem and progenitor cells (HSC/HPC), lymphocytes, monocytes, and mesenchymal stromal cells (MSC). Myeloid and red blood cells (RBCs) are typically excluded by the process of separating BMMNC from the bone marrow aspirate.

Subsequent studies have further characterized more specific subsets of angiogenic stem and progenitor populations in the BMMNC fraction. Asahara et al. have shown that circulating mononuclear cells expressing CD34 or Flk-1 could differentiate into endothelial cells in vitro and contribute to vasculogenesis in vivo in adult animals, thus they were identified as putative endothelial progenitor cells (EPC) [1]. Kamihata et al. further demonstrated that BMMNC contain EPC in the CD34+ cell fraction and proangiogenic factor-producing cells in the CD34− cell fraction. The CD34+ BMMNC more actively form cord-like structures by coculture with CD34- BMMNC, suggesting a synergy between these two fractions to enhance the angiogenesis process [2]. The CD34+ cells, consisting of mostly hematopoietic stem and progenitor cells, can also be mobilized to peripheral blood by systemic injection of G-CSF, and these CD34+ peripheral blood mononuclear cells (PBMNC) can then be harvested for therapeutic angiogenesis.

Regenerative Medicine for Peripheral Artery Disease. http://dx.doi.org/10.1016/B978-0-12-801344-1.00003-6

It is worth noting that with more extensive efforts invested on isolating putative EPC from peripheral blood or bone marrow, the concept of EPC has become progressively sophisticated and controversial, as different groups have used different terms to describe "EPC"-like cells by different identification and isolation methods. These terms include but are not limited to colony forming unit of endothelial cells (CFU-EC) [3,4], circulating angiogenic cells (CAC) [5], culture-expanded endothelial progenitor cells (CE-EPC) [6], culture-modified mononuclear cells (CMMC) [7], endothelial outgrowth cells (EOC) [8], endothelial progenitor-derived cells (EPDC) [9], circulating endothelial cells (CEC) [10], circulating endothelial progenitors (CEP) [11], and endothelial colony forming cells (ECFC) [12]. Despite these long-standing controversies, it has been increasingly recognized that many markers previously used to identify putative EPC such as CD34, CD117, and CD133 are shared by myeloid cells of various stages of differentiation [13,14]. Thus the boundary between EPC and myeloid derivatives is vague, if not completely nonexistent [15].

Aldehyde dehydrogenase (ALDH) is a cytosolic enzyme responsible for oxidizing a variety of aldehydes including vitamin A [16]. ALDH is expressed at high levels in hematopoietic stem and progenitors (HSC/HPC) and is responsible for the resistance of HSC/HPC to the inhibitory effects of alkylating agents such as cyclophosphamide and 4-hydroxyperoxycyclophosphamide on cell proliferation [17–19]. Using fluorescent substrate for ALDH, such as BODIPY aminoacetaldehyde (BAAA), HSC/HPC can be fluorescently labeled and enriched through flow cytometry [20]. Capoccia et al. purified primitive HSC/HPC from human bone marrow by selection of cells with high ALDH activity. After intravenous injection into immune-deficient mice with hindlimb ischemia (HLI), these cells significantly increased recovery of blood perfusion and capillary density in the ischemic limb. Flow cytometry analysis showed that ALDH activity-high cells contain a much higher concentration of CD34 + CD133 + CD14 + CD117 (c-Kit)+ cells compared to those with low ALDH activity [21].

Another important subset of BMMNC is MSC. The MSCs are characterized by their adherence to plastic surface and abilities to self-renew and, in permissive cultures, differentiate into osteocytes, chondrocytes, and adipocytes [22]. Although extremely rare in the bone marrow (~1 in every 100,000 total bone marrow cells), these cells can be expanded ex vivo to larger quantities to achieve desirable dosage for therapeutic use [23]. A dedicated chapter with more thorough introduction of BMMSC in the context of peripheral arterial disease is also included in this book.

Isolation of BMMNC

BMMNC used for peripheral arterial disease (PAD) patients in clinical trials are typically aspirated from the ileum under local anaesthesia, purified and concentrated to a final volume of about 40–50 mL and then delivered back to patients either by intramuscular injection into the gastrocnemius and foot of the ischemic leg or by intraarterial injection through catheter [24,25].

The purification step was initially accomplished using Ficoll™ density-gradient centrifugation system with slight variations by different groups [26,27]. Such technique requires a good clinical practice (GCP)-certified facility for bone marrow processing, and sterile-cell biology laboratory if cell culture and expansion is warranted. Furthermore, purity of the BMMNC has significant clinical implications in therapeutic applications. In a study using BMMNC for the treatment of ST-elevation myocardial infarction, although standard density gradient centrifugation method with lymphocyte separation medium (Lonza) was used, nearly 0.2×10^9 residual RBCs were still present in the 200 million BMMNC and 36% of the BMMNC were neutrophils. Notably, when the amount of contaminated RBC in the BMMNC exceeds 0.4×10^9/200 million BMMNC, it is inversely correlated with the recovery of left ventricular ejection fraction (LVEF), whereas no significant association was detected for the number of contaminating neutrophils [28].

For more practical purposes, several point-of-care, bedside, closed systems have been developed to streamline the process from bone marrow aspiration to final cell-product generation. Examples of these devices include MarrowStim™ system from Biomet Inc. and SmartPrep system from Harvest Technologies. These new isolation techniques were able to achieve similar yield of progenitor cells compared to conventional density-gradient-based method; meanwhile they substantially shortened the therapy time and saved the cost of laboratory facilities previously required for cell processing [29,30]. Pilot experiments in a mouse model of HLI demonstrated that the angiogenic potency of the bone marrow cell products from point-of-care device was at least equivalent, if not higher than that of BMMNC obtained through the Ficoll isolation procedure [31].

In preclinical studies, especially in rodents, BMMNC harvest requires sacrificing the donor and flushing long bones (ie, femur and tibia) to obtain total bone marrow cells. Further purification of BMMNC is achieved by lysis of RBCs and density-gradient centrifugation with Ficoll™ solution.

PRECLINICAL EVIDENCE FOR BMMNC BENEFITS IN PAD

Animal models of HLI to mimic human peripheral arterial disease have been developed in several animal species. The rodent model is the most commonly used, although HLI in other animal species such as rabbit, porcine, canine, and primate have also been described [32–35]. The advantage of rodent models is obvious, they allow larger number of experimental replications, lower per animal cost, and modifiable genetic background. That said, larger animal models have their unique merits including closer resemblance of human vascular wall structure and hemodynamics, and easier access to individual blood vessels [36].

Lawall et al. provided an excellent review of animal models of HLI, using species including rabbit, rat, and mouse, in which BMMNC or subsets of

BMMNC, including EPC and MSC, were tested and showed promising effects of these cells to promote blood perfusion, increase capillary density and homing of EPC, upregulate local VEGF and b-FGF levels, and decrease autoamputation rate and muscle atrophy [37].

In most of these studies, improvement of blood flow in the distal limb reflected enhanced angiogenesis as documented by laser Doppler perfusion imaging. A more definitive method to quantify capillary density within the gastrocnemius or soleus muscles is the technique of immunohistochemical (IHC) staining for the endothelial cell marker such CD31. This is a labor-intensive process and capillary formation requires correlation with the perfusion indices previously described. Additional methods to assess limb perfusion have also been developed in recent years, including arterial flow probes, microspheres, contrast-enhanced direct injection X-ray, MRI angiography, micro-CT, and contrast-enhanced ultrasound sonography (CEUS), each with unique advantages, beyond the scope of this review, and summarized by Lotfi et al. [38].

In addition to blood perfusion, other endpoints in the animal models of CLI can also be measured to evaluate the efficacy of progenitor cells, such as exercise tolerance, tissue necrosis, and functional recovery from claudication [39,40]. The most reproducible measure of therapeutic intervention in CLI is tissue necrosis. In BALB/c mice, for instance, the degree of distal limb necrosis after femoral artery ligation could be scored from 1 to 5 to allow quantitative comparisons between individual animals. The caveat with tissue necrosis as an endpoint, however, is that individual responses to femoral artery ligation may vary dramatically between different strains or even within the same strain of mice, most likely due to the inter- and intrastrain differences in collateralization [41]. Therefore, larger size of treatment groups is often necessary in the experimental design to assure sufficient statistical power.

Despite the extensive use of HLI as an in vivo angiogenesis assay to evaluate the efficacy of novel proangiogenic agents, its value as a preclinical model to represent the pathogenesis of PAD is still highly controversial. Although this in vivo assay incorporates the dynamics between endothelial cells, smooth muscle cells, pericytes, and leukocytes in the complicated process of neovascularization well beyond any 2-D in vitro assays with only selected cell types, several key differences between HLI mice and PAD patients must be recognized. In an HLI model, arterial occlusion is induced acutely by ligation or cauterization of femoral artery, whereas human PAD develops chronically as a consequence of atherosclerosis and is often accompanied by the presence of thrombosis. In addition, mice used for HLI model are young and healthy, whereas PAD patients usually present with advanced age and multiple comorbidities such as diabetes, hypertension, and hyperlipidemia. Therefore, it is not surprising that agents showing consistent promising effects in rodent models of HLI, such as VEGF, FGF, and HGF, only yield mixed results in human clinical trials. Although HGF showed most promising effects on improving rest pain and quality of life scores in a randomized, double-blind, placebo-controlled clinical trial, gene therapies based on VEGF and FGF have failed to improve the designed primary endpoints, such as rate of amputation events, or time to major amputation or death [42–45].

POTENTIAL MECHANISMS OF BMMNC IN PAD

Reconstruction of Vascular Endothelial Architecture

The highly heterogeneous composition of BMMNC provides a complex source of various adult stem and progenitor cell types for cell replacement and regeneration at the injury site, and complicates definitive description of mechanisms of these cells. Using multiple physiological and pathological neovascularization models, Asahara et al. demonstrated that progenitor cells can be mobilized from bone marrow to incorporate into the newly formed capillaries and contribute to the new vascular structure [46,47]. These mobilized CD34+ mononuclear cells have been recognized as putative EPCs because of their apparent ability to differentiate into endothelial cells producing nitric oxide in response to EC-dependent agonist acetylcholine and the EC-specific mitogen VEGF [1]. This observation is echoed by the studies of angiogenesis in the context of tumor growth, as several groups reported bone marrow-derived cells being recruited and incorporated into the vascular architecture of tumor vessels and exhibited phenotypes of endothelial cells [48].

Although incorporation of bone marrow-derived HSC in the neovasculature was initially accepted, the extent of such incorporation has progressively become controversial, as expression of endothelial cell markers such as von Willebrand factor seems to be rare or even absent in several studies, whereas in other studies GFP-labeled bone marrow–derived cells were not detected in the vessel wall at all.

Stabilization of Neovasculature via Pericyte Differentiation

Pericytes are polymorphic, multibranched cells located within the basement membrane of capillary and postcapillary venules with envelopment of endothelial cells. Pericytes play a critical role in stabilizing vascular wall, controlling endothelial cell proliferation, and regulating microvascular blood flow [49]. In the process of neovascular sprouting, pericytes provide both prosurvival signaling and mechanical support to maintain the newly formed endothelium via the direct interactions with endothelial cells [50]. Rajantie et al. created bone marrow GFP+ chimeric mice and showed that bone marrow–derived endothelial cells do not significantly contribute to tumor- or cytokine-induced angiogenesis. Instead, bone marrow–derived pericytes were persistently detected at sites of tumor-induced or vascular endothelial growth factor–induced angiogenesis [51]. Similarly, Ziegelhoeffer et al. also used GFP+ chimeric mice to look into the involvement of bone marrow–derived GFP+ cells in the postischemic angiogenesis process in a mouse CLI model. They were not able to colocalize GFP signals with endothelial or smooth muscle cell markers, suggesting lack of direct structural contribution from bone marrow cells to the neovasculature. Instead, ample GFP+ cells were found in the perivascular space resembling fibroblasts and pericytes based on their shape and distribution [52]. Such specific recruitment of bone marrow–derived pericyte precursors was also observed in the process of corneal vasculogenesis [53]. Notably, over 90% of the bone marrow–derived pericytes, as defined by their expression of nerve/glial antigen-2 (NG2) and platelet-derived growth factor receptor β (PDGF-β) receptor, also express CD45 and CD11b, suggesting their hematopoietic origin from the bone marrow.

Secretion of Proangiogenic Factors

In addition to direct incorporation into vascular structure, BMMNC also exhibited potent paracrine activities to secrete proangiogenic factors to further promote angiogenesis [54]. Such proangiogenic nature seems to be shared by almost all subsets of BMMNC, including HSC and EPC, although the specific cytokines being secreted may vary between cell types [5,55]. Such mutual complementation may explain the synergy between different subsets of BMMNC. For example, Kamihata et al. demonstrated that CD34-negative fraction of BMMNC secrete basic fibroblast growth factor (bFGF), vascular endothelial growth factor (VEGF), and angiopoietin 1 (Ang 1); and that CD34-positive cells from peripheral or cord blood may be induced to form more abundant cord-like structures by coculture with CD34-negative fraction [2]. It is worth noting that the more mature cellular components are also critical parts of the BMMNC cocktail, which include T lymphocytes, megakaryocytes, platelets, and monocytes [56–59]. For instance, CD4–/– mice showed reduced collateral flow induction and vascular endothelial growth factor levels in the ischemic muscle compared with wild-type mice, and consequently delayed recovery of hindlimb function and increased muscle atrophy/fibrosis, which was significantly improved following reinfusion of purified CD4+ T cells [56].

Among the heterogeneous composition of BMMNC, mesenchymal stromal cells are of particular interest. This unique population of cells are capable of secreting a broad spectrum of chemokines, cytokines, and proangiogenic factors [60]. Furthermore, it has been increasingly recognized that their paracrine functions are highly adaptive to the microenvironment signals by changing the level and composition of trophic factors secreted [61,62]. It is therefore not surprising that the conditioned medium generated from MSC contains such a rich mixture of key trophic factors that it can, in the absence of producer cells, promote proliferation and migration of endothelial cells and vascular smooth muscle cells in vitro, and enhances blood flow recovery of ischemic hindlimb in vivo [39,60,63,64]. This could translate into a significant advancement in the stem-cell therapy and allow more stringent quality-control procedures and larger-scale manufacturing of highly reproducible "off-the-shelf" cellular products for the same indications currently showing promising benefits from stem-cell therapy.

CLINICAL TRIALS USING BMMNC FOR CLI PATIENTS

Overview of BMMNC in CLI

In light of promising effect of BMMNC to promote neovascularization in the animal models of HLI, the earliest human clinical trial was initiated even while studies on the mechanisms of BMMNC to address ischemic diseases were still unfolding. In 2002, Tateishi-Yuyama et al. published the first large clinical trial using intramuscular injections of autologous BMMNC for PAD patients with CLI (therapeutic angiogenesis using cell transplantation, TACT) [24]. In this study, 25 patients with unilateral limb ischemia received intramuscular injection of BMMNC ($1.6 \pm 0.6 \times 10^9$ cells) into the gastrocnemius of the ischemic limb (ankle-brachial index, ABI < 0.6). The contralateral less ischemic limb (ABI > 0.6) received saline injection as a control. No adverse events related to treatment were reported, and BMMNC administration improved subjects' ABI, transcutaneous oxygen pressure ($TcPO_2$), rest pain, and pain-free walking distance at 4 and 24 weeks. The same study also recruited 22 patients with bilateral limb ischemia. Each subject randomly received BMMNC injection into one limb as active treatment and PBMNC into the other limb as a control. Compared to PBMNC, BMMNC significantly improved ABI, $TcPO_2$, rest pain, and pain-free walking time at 4 and 24 weeks.

The encouraging results from TACT study inspired more clinical trials in different countries on the efficacy of BMMNC in improving limb salvage in patients with CLI, including the first phase-I/II clinical trial approved by FDA and conducted by our group in the United States [65]. In this open-label trial, a total of 29 patients (30 limbs treated) between the ages of 23 and 84 with CLI defined as symptoms of rest pain and/or ulceration with an ABI ≤ 0.55 and/or toe brachial index (TBI) ≤ 0.40 were enrolled. Enrolled patients had no patent artery below the knee that was continuous to the foot and thus no options for bypass and/or endovascular approaches to improving perfusion, as determined by an independent vascular surgeon. Ficoll density centrifugation (FC) was used to isolate BMMNC for the first 14 patients and MarrowStim™ (MS) closed centrifugation system was used for the other 15 patients. The average number of cells injected was $1.3 \pm 0.7 \times 10^9$ using FC method and $2.0 \pm 1.6 \times 10^9$ using MS method. Among these 29 patients, the amputation-free survival (AFS) at 1 year was 86.3%, which is much higher than AFS at 1 year reported in other studies [30,66]. There was a significant increase from baseline in first toe pressure (FTP) by 10.2 ± 6.2 mmHg ($p = 0.02$) and in TBI by $0.10 + 0.05$ ($p = 0.02$) at week 12. Rest pain decreased significantly at 12 weeks from baseline. The VascuQol total score increased in all categories, especially in the domains of emotion (2.5 ± 0.3 to 4.3 ± 0.5) and pain (2.5 ± 0.4 to 4.0 ± 0.7). Three of nine ulcers (33%) healed completely by week 12. There were two procedure-related serious adverse events (SAEs)—anemia-related myocardial ischemia and entrapment of a guidewire during contrast arteriography, which was initially used to assess efficacy of cell therapy. Similar CLI studies have also reported reduction of hematocrit in patients after large volume bone marrow aspiration, however, it was transient and well tolerated without any need for interventions [67].

Since the TACT study in 2002, clinical studies on BMMNC therapy in PAD patients have advanced from early small-scale, uncontrolled phase-I trials to randomized, controlled, phase-III clinical trials. A recent metaanalysis published in 2013 selected studies that are randomized and controlled, involve bone marrow–derived cells, have a comparator group, and have endpoints such as major amputation, survival, ABI, $PTcO_2$, pain score, pain-free walking distance. The exclusion criteria include studies performed in children or neonates, animal studies, review or case reports ($n < 10$), no CLI or diabetic foot, not published in English, Dutch, or German, gene therapy, diagnostic, prognostic, or etiologic studies. This selection strategy resulted in inclusion of 12 RCT using bone marrow–derived cells, including BMMNC, BMMSC, PBMNC, and Ixmyelocel-T cells [68]. Six out of these twelve RCTs used only BMMNC and were summarized in Table 3.1.

Safety of BMMNC in CLI

The procedure of bone marrow aspiration and injection of BMMNC has generally proven free from serious adverse events and safe in patients with CLI. Bone marrow aspiration has been reported to result in a mean decrease in hematocrit

TABLE 3.1 Randomized Controlled Trials of BMMNC for CLI

References	Sample size	Cell number (10^9)	Route	Follow-up (months)	Outcome
[69]	13/12	1–3	IM	4	Improved ABI, $TcPO_2$, rest pain, pain-free walking distance, ulcer healing
[67]	34/14	240 mL	IM	24	No change in ABI or AFS
[77]	21/41 limbs	0.93	IM	24	Improved ABI, $TcPO_2$, pain-free walking time, ulcer healing
[29]	42/54	240 mL	IM	16	Decreased amputation rate
[24]	22/22 limbs	0.88–2.8	IM	24	Improved ABI, $TcPO_2$, rest pain, pain-free walking time
[25]	19/21	0.15	IA	72	Improved pain score, ulcer healing

Sample size: treatment group/control group; *ABI*, ankle brachial index; *$TcPO_2$*, transcutaneous O_2 pressure; *AFS*, amputation free survival; *IM*, intramuscular; *IA*, intraarterial.

by 2.6% as compared to controls, which is well tolerated in most patients, however it may pose a risk to those who are anemic at baseline and have coronary artery disease [67]. In our experience, we have addressed this issue by adjusting the volume of bone marrow aspirated for patients with preexisting cardiovascular conditions to minimize risk of ischemic events [65]. No muscular damage (elevation in creatinine phosphokinase), vascular malformation, or acute renal injury has been associated with intramuscular injection of BMMNC. For delivery of BMMNC through catheter (intraarterial injection), three procedure-related adverse events were reported, including stent thrombosis, hematoma in the groin, and a pseudoaneurysm, all resolved without sequelae [25].

To assess the long-term safety of BMMNC therapy, Matoba et al. followed up patients from the TACT study for 3 years. The 3-year overall survival rates were 80% (95% CI 68–91) in patients with atherosclerotic peripheral arterial disease (11 deaths in 74 patients) and 100% in 41 patients with thromboangiitis obliterans [70]. Another study (BONMOT-1) followed 51 patients for 3.2 years and reported limb salvage rate of 59% at 6 months and 53% at last follow-up. No unexpected long-term adverse events were reported [30].

Primary Endpoints for BMMNC in CLI

The most widely accepted primary outcomes to evaluate the efficacy of therapeutic agents for CLI patients are major amputation rates and AFS, a composite of major amputation and all-cause mortality [71]. Benoit et al. conducted a double-blinded randomized controlled trial (RCT) evaluating the efficacy of concentrated bone marrow cells (BMAC) in 48 no-option CLI patients. At the 6-month follow-up, patients with tissue loss and those treated with BMAC demonstrated a lower amputation rate than placebo (39.1% vs 71.4%, $p = 0.1337$). The Kaplan–Meier time to amputation was longer in the BMAC group than in the placebo group ($p = 0.067$). Based on a bootstrap simulation model, in order to detect significant difference in AFS between BMAC and placebo with a power of 95%, a sample size of 210 patients would be required, which is very difficult to achieve in a single-site clinical trial [67]. A recent metaanalysis incorporating results from 9 RCTs compared the aggregate of the therapeutic groups with 259 limbs and the control groups with 232 limbs. The results showed that bone marrow–derived cell therapy significantly reduced major amputation rates compared with the placebo control, with a RR of 0.58 (95%CI, 0.40–0.84; $p = 0.004$). The corresponding absolute risk reduction is 12.1% and the number needed to treat to prevent 1 major amputation is 8. Conventional surgical revascularization, such as prosthetic femorotibial bypass, which achieves limb salvage rates of 72.5% at 1 year and 61.9% at 5 years [72]. Although the improvement from cell therapy is limited compared to surgery, considering the high morbidity, long hospital stay, requirement of intensive care unit, association with surgery, this safe and minimally invasive novel therapy still offers a very promising treatment modality for CLI patients, especially those considered having no-option or those who have poor options—prosthetic or composite graft required for revascularization. There is also a promising trend of increasing AFS in the cell-therapy group compared to the control with a RR of 1.16 (95%CI 0.92–1.48) but this did not reach statistical significance. This is probably because the calculation of RR for AFS was performed using data from 6 out of these 9 RCT (no AFS data 3 out of 9 studies), which reduced the sample size in the cell-therapy group from 234 to 157 limbs. As mentioned previously, this did not meet the sample size requirement of 210 patients to detect any difference in AFS between the cell-treatment group and the control [73].

Secondary Endpoints for BMMNC in CLI

Functional endpoints such as pain-free walking distance/time, pain score, ulcer healing, and quality of life survey have often been used as secondary outcomes, especially in small-scale phase-I/II clinical trials. These endpoints have shown significant improvement after bone marrow cell therapy across numerous studies. A metaanalysis of 8 RCTs with 237 limbs showed an overall RR of complete ulcer healing of 1.87 (95% CI, 1.49–2.36; $p < 0.00001$) in the bone marrow cell treatment group; Similarly, pain score in the therapeutic arm was 1.10 (95% CI, 1.37– 0.83; $p < 0.00001$) based on 8 RCT, and pain-free walking distance was substantially longer in the therapeutic arm based on 3 RCT [73]. The caveat with functional endpoints is that their accuracy in evaluating true efficacy of test therapy is often hampered by the subjectivity of the patient and investigator, especially when invasive procedures such as bone marrow aspirations are involved.

Other commonly used secondary outcomes include physiological measurements, such as ABI, TBI, FTP, and $TcPO_2$. Metaanalysis of 7 RCT showed that ABI was significantly improved by 0.12 (95% CI, 0.09 – 0.15, $p < 0.00001$) and $TcPO_2$ was significantly increased by 14.28 mmHg (95%CI, 8.54–20.02; $p < 0.00001$) following bone marrow–derived cell treatment [73]. However, the enthusiasm over improvements in these endpoints was dampened by the controversies over the correlation between vascular patency and long-term outcome of patients. Moreover, bone marrow cell therapy has been shown to mostly improve microvascular sprouting and formation; therefore, the causal relationship between cell injection and improvement of ABI which reflects blood flow in large vessels is unclear.

CLINICAL TRIALS USING SUBSETS OF BMMNC FOR CLI PATIENTS

Although most clinical trials have been using BMMNC, other bone marrow–derived cell subsets have been increasingly explored in recent clinical trials. Peripheral blood mononuclear cells mobilized by granulocyte colony-stimulating factor (G-CSF) are a commonly used substitute to avoid bone marrow aspiration. This procedure requires 6 days of treatment with G-CSF, after which the PBMNC are harvested by apheresis for autologous injection. In a controlled trial, Huang et al. reported that 3 months after receiving PBMNC, patients showed significant improvement in limb pain, ulcer healing, and ABI, compared to those receiving the placebo control [74]. This result has been further confirmed by two subsequent RCTs also using PBMNC. Ozturk et al. reported improved ABI and pain score in the PBMNC treatment group [75]. Mohammadzadeh et al. reported improved ABI and decreased amputation rates as a result of PBMNC treatment [76].

Bone marrow mesenchymal stromal cells (BMMSC) are another promising subpopulation of bone marrow cells receiving increasing attention. There are three advantages of BMMSC: (1) they can be expanded ex vivo to larger quantities and therefore require much smaller volume of bone marrow aspiration; (2) BMMSC are immunomodulatory in a manner which may facilitate allogeneic transplantation of cells from younger and healthier donors, as well as industrial manufacturing of "off-the-shelf" cellular products; (3) they are purer and more defined than BMMNC and can be tested in preclinical models for potency before applying to patients. Lu et al. conducted an RCT to compare BMMSC with BMMNC in CLI patients with bilateral limb ischemia. Only 30 mL bone marrow was aspirated from the BMMSC group and BMMSC were isolated and expanded in vitro to reach target dosage; 300 mL bone marrow was aspirated from the BMMNC group. By 24 weeks, BMMSC and BMMNC both significantly improved ABI, $TcPO_2$, and pain-free walking time, compared to placebo control. MRA-based collateral-blood-vessel scores were significantly higher and the ulcer healing was faster in the BMMSC group [77]. Gupta tested safety and efficacy of allogeneic BMMSC versus placebo in 20 CLI patients. At 6-month follow-up, ABI was improved significantly in the BMMSC by an average of 0.22 ($p = 0.0018$). No adverse events were associated with BMMSC treatment [78].

A variety of other cell types have also been under active investigation in PAD patients, including CD34 + PBMNC [79,80], ALDH+ BMMNC [81], and Ixmyelocel-T [82]. Most studies for these cell types are still in phase-I/II stage. Their efficacy for CLI patients are yet to be tested in larger phase-III clinical trials.

CONCLUSIONS AND FUTURE DIRECTIONS

BMMNC represent a mixture of angiogenic stem and progenitor cells, as well as mature hematopoietic cells that function synergistically to promote neovascularization. Delivery of BMMNC or its subpopulations have demonstrated marked effects of these cells to improve revascularization of ischemic tissue in preclinical models, such as murine models of HLI. Extensive phase-I and phase-II clinical trials in human PAD patients have established the safety of BMMNC and showed promising effects of the cells to improve ischemic pain, ulcer size, pain-free walking distance, ABI, and $TcPO_2$. However, the ability to determine the efficacy of BMMNC on major amputation rates, AFS, or all-cause mortality is limited by the absence of phase-III pivotal RCTs, disparity in cell doses used, and method of delivery in smaller phase-II studies. Furthermore, the heterogeneity of the CLI patient population, which includes atherosclerosis, thromboangitis obliterans, and premature diabetic medial calcinosis of the tibial and peroneal arteries, confounds the ability to determine the ideal patient population for BMMNC therapy.

Future larger placebo-controlled RCTs are clearly warranted before any decisions on translating BMMNC therapy to standard care of advanced PAD patients can be made. As part of the effort, we will complete enrollment of 152 patients with CLI in the first randomized, placebo controlled phase-III trial in May 2015 in the United States that will determine efficacy of BMMNC in promoting freedom from AFS. This study will be pivotal in the field as it will be the largest RCT to date and will be including ancillary studies to delineate the mechanisms by which BMMNC may improve perfusion and promote limb salvage. In addition, we anticipate that this trial will provide a demographic and genomic signature of patients who best respond to BMMNC treatment. Of equally critical importance are clinical studies designed to optimize the BMMNC therapy through multidosing comparisons, enhance BMMNC survival with adjunctive biomatrices, and precondition cells with treatment such as hypoxia to maximize the performance of cells in vivo.

REFERENCES

[1] Asahara T, et al. Isolation of putative progenitor endothelial cells for angiogenesis. Science 1997;275:964–7.
[2] Kamihata H, et al. Implantation of bone marrow mononuclear cells into ischemic myocardium enhances collateral perfusion and regional function via side supply of angioblasts, angiogenic ligands, and cytokines. Circulation 2001;104:1046–52.
[3] Gehling UM, et al. In vitro differentiation of endothelial cells from AC133-positive progenitor cells. Blood 2000;95:3106–12.
[4] Hill JM, et al. Circulating endothelial progenitor cells, vascular function, and cardiovascular risk. N Engl J Med 2003;348:593–600.
[5] Rehman J, Li J, Orschell CM, March KL. Peripheral blood "endothelial progenitor cells" are derived from monocyte/macrophages and secrete angiogenic growth factors. Circulation 2003;107:1164–9.
[6] Sharpe EE 3rd, et al. The origin and in vivo significance of murine and human culture-expanded endothelial progenitor cells. Am J Pathol 2006;168:1710–21.
[7] Gulati R, et al. Autologous culture-modified mononuclear cells confer vascular protection after arterial injury. Circulation 2003;108:1520–6.
[8] Lin Y, Weisdorf DJ, Solovey A, Hebbel RP. Origins of circulating endothelial cells and endothelial outgrowth from blood. J Clin Invest 2000;105:71–7.
[9] Bompais H, et al. Human endothelial cells derived from circulating progenitors display specific functional properties compared with mature vessel wall endothelial cells. Blood 2004;103:2577–84.

[10] Lin Y, et al. Use of blood outgrowth endothelial cells for gene therapy for hemophilia A. Blood 2002;99:457–62.

[11] Romagnani P, et al. CD14+CD34low cells with stem cell phenotypic and functional features are the major source of circulating endothelial progenitors. Circ Res 2005;97:314–22.

[12] Ingram DA, et al. Identification of a novel hierarchy of endothelial progenitor cells using human peripheral and umbilical cord blood. Blood 2004;104:2752–60.

[13] Fadini GP, Losordo D, Dimmeler S. Critical reevaluation of endothelial progenitor cell phenotypes for therapeutic and diagnostic use. Circ Res 2012;110:624–37.

[14] Yoder MC. Human endothelial progenitor cells. CSH Perspect Med 2012;2. a006692.

[15] Yoder MC. Endothelial progenitor cell: a blood cell by many other names may serve similar functions. J Mol Med 2013;91:285–95.

[16] Labrecque J, Bhat PV, Lacroix A. Purification and partial characterization of a rat kidney aldehyde dehydrogenase that oxidizes retinal to retinoic acid. Biochem Cell Biol 1993;71:85–9.

[17] Gordon MY, Goldman JM, Gordon-Smith EC. 4-Hydroperoxycyclophosphamide inhibits proliferation by human granulocyte-macrophage colony-forming cells (GM-CFC) but spares more primitive progenitor cells. Leukemia Res 1985;9:1017–21.

[18] Sahovic EA, Colvin M, Hilton J, Ogawa M. Role for aldehyde dehydrogenase in survival of progenitors for murine blast cell colonies after treatment with 4-hydroperoxycyclophosphamide in vitro. Cancer Res 1988;48:1223–6.

[19] Smith C, et al. Purification and partial characterization of a human hematopoietic precursor population. Blood 1991;77:2122–8.

[20] Storms RW, et al. Isolation of primitive human hematopoietic progenitors on the basis of aldehyde dehydrogenase activity. Proc Natl Acad Sci USA 1999;96:9118–23.

[21] Capoccia BJ, et al. Revascularization of ischemic limbs after transplantation of human bone marrow cells with high aldehyde dehydrogenase activity. Blood 2009;113:5340–51.

[22] Pittenger MF, et al. Multilineage potential of adult human mesenchymal stem cells. Science 1999;284:143–7.

[23] Thirumala S, Goebel WS, Woods EJ. Manufacturing and banking of mesenchymal stem cells. Expert Opin Biol Ther 2013;13:673–91.

[24] Tateishi-Yuyama E, et al. Therapeutic angiogenesis for patients with limb ischaemia by autologous transplantation of bone-marrow cells: a pilot study and a randomised controlled trial. Lancet 2002;360:427–35.

[25] Walter DH, et al. Intraarterial administration of bone marrow mononuclear cells in patients with critical limb ischemia: a randomized-start, placebo-controlled pilot trial (PROVASA). Circulation 2011;4:26–37.

[26] Boyum A. Separation of lymphocytes, lymphocyte subgroups and monocytes: a review. Lymphology 1977;10:71–6.

[27] Boyum A, Brincker Fjerdingstad H, Martinsen I, Lea T, Lovhaug D. Separation of human lymphocytes from citrated blood by density gradient (NycoPrep) centrifugation: monocyte depletion depending upon activation of membrane potassium channels. Scandinavian J Immunol 2002;56:76–84.

[28] Assmus B, et al. Red blood cell contamination of the final cell product impairs the efficacy of autologous bone marrow mononuclear cell therapy. J Am Coll Cardiol 2010;55:1385–94.

[29] Prochazka V, et al. Autologous bone marrow stem cell transplantation in patients with end-stage chronical critical limb ischemia and diabetic foot. Vnitrni lekarstvi 2009;55:173–8.

[30] Amann B, Luedemann C, Ratei R, Schmidt-Lucke JA. Autologous bone marrow cell transplantation increases leg perfusion and reduces amputations in patients with advanced critical limb ischemia due to peripheral artery disease. Cell Transplant 2009;18:371–80.

[31] Hermann PC, et al. Concentration of bone marrow total nucleated cells by a point-of-care device provides a high yield and preserves their functional activity. Cell Transplant 2008;16:1059–69.
[32] Burkhardt GE, et al. A large animal survival model (Sus scrofa) of extremity ischemia/reperfusion and neuromuscular outcomes assessment: a pilot study. J Trauma 2010;69(Suppl 1):S146–53.
[33] Nakada MT, et al. Clot lysis in a primate model of peripheral arterial occlusive disease with use of systemic or intraarterial reteplase: addition of abciximab results in improved vessel reperfusion. J Vasc Interv Radiol 2004;15:169–76.
[34] Arras M, et al. Monocyte activation in angiogenesis and collateral growth in the rabbit hindlimb. J Clin Invest 1998;101:40–50.
[35] Rosenthal SL, Guyton AC. Hemodynamics of collateral vasodilatation following femoral artery occlusion in anesthetized dogs. Circ Res 1968;23:239–48.
[36] Madeddu P, et al. Murine models of myocardial and limb ischemia: diagnostic end-points and relevance to clinical problems. Vascular Pharmacol 2006;45:281–301.
[37] Lawall H, Bramlage P, Amann B. Stem cell and progenitor cell therapy in peripheral artery disease. A critical appraisal. Thromb Haemost 2010;103:696–709.
[38] Lotfi S, et al. Towards a more relevant hind limb model of muscle ischaemia. Atherosclerosis 2013;227:1–8.
[39] Kinnaird T, et al. Local delivery of marrow-derived stromal cells augments collateral perfusion through paracrine mechanisms. Circulation 2004;109:1543–9.
[40] Helisch A, et al. Impact of mouse strain differences in innate hindlimb collateral vasculature. Arterioscl Throm Vas 2006;26:520–6.
[41] Dokun AO, et al. A quantitative trait locus (LSq-1) on mouse chromosome 7 is linked to the absence of tissue loss after surgical hindlimb ischemia. Circulation 2008;117:1207–15.
[42] Becit N, et al. The effect of vascular endothelial growth factor on angiogenesis: an experimental study. Eur J Vasc Endovasc Surg 2001;22:310–6.
[43] Mac Gabhann F, Qutub AA, Annex BH, Popel AS. Systems biology of pro-angiogenic therapies targeting the VEGF system. Wiley Interdiscip Rev 2010;2:694–707.
[44] Belch J, et al. Effect of fibroblast growth factor NV1FGF on amputation and death: a randomised placebo-controlled trial of gene therapy in critical limb ischaemia. Lancet 2011;377:1929–37.
[45] Shigematsu H, et al. Randomized, double-blind, placebo-controlled clinical trial of hepatocyte growth factor plasmid for critical limb ischemia. Gene Ther 2010;17:1152–61.
[46] Asahara T, et al. Bone marrow origin of endothelial progenitor cells responsible for postnatal vasculogenesis in physiological and pathological neovascularization. Circ Res 1999;85:221–8.
[47] Takahashi T, et al. Ischemia- and cytokine-induced mobilization of bone marrow-derived endothelial progenitor cells for neovascularization. Nat Med 1999;5:434–8.
[48] Santarelli JG, et al. Incorporation of bone marrow-derived Flk-1-expressing CD34+ cells in the endothelium of tumor vessels in the mouse brain. Neurosurgery 2006;59:374–82.
[49] Ribatti D, Nico B, Crivellato E. The role of pericytes in angiogenesis. Int J Dev Biol 2011;55:261–8.
[50] Hall AP. Review of the pericyte during angiogenesis and its role in cancer and diabetic retinopathy. Toxicol Pathol 2006;34:763–75.
[51] Rajantie I, et al. Adult bone marrow-derived cells recruited during angiogenesis comprise precursors for periendothelial vascular mural cells. Blood 2004;104:2084–6.

[52] Ziegelhoeffer T, et al. Bone marrow-derived cells do not incorporate into the adult growing vasculature. Circ Res 2004;94:230–8.

[53] Ozerdem U, Alitalo K, Salven P, Li A. Contribution of bone marrow-derived pericyte precursor cells to corneal vasculogenesis. Invest Ophthalmol Vis Sci 2005;46:3502–6.

[54] Fuchs S, et al. Transendocardial delivery of autologous bone marrow enhances collateral perfusion and regional function in pigs with chronic experimental myocardial ischemia. J Am Coll Cardiol 2001;37:1726–32.

[55] Jackson KA, et al. Regeneration of ischemic cardiac muscle and vascular endothelium by adult stem cells. J Clin Invest 2001;107:1395–402.

[56] Stabile E, et al. Impaired arteriogenic response to acute hindlimb ischemia in CD4-knockout mice. Circulation 2003;108:205–10.

[57] Mohle R, Green D, Moore MA, Nachman RL, Rafii S. Constitutive production and thrombin-induced release of vascular endothelial growth factor by human megakaryocytes and platelets. Proc Natl Acad Sci USA 1997;94:663–8.

[58] Blotnick S, Peoples GE, Freeman MR, Eberlein TJ, Klagsbrun M. T lymphocytes synthesize and export heparin-binding epidermal growth factor-like growth factor and basic fibroblast growth factor, mitogens for vascular cells and fibroblasts: differential production and release by CD4+ and CD8+ T cells. Proc Natl Acad Sci USA 1994;91:2890–4.

[59] Melter M, et al. Ligation of CD40 induces the expression of vascular endothelial growth factor by endothelial cells and monocytes and promotes angiogenesis in vivo. Blood 2000;96:3801–8.

[60] Kinnaird T, et al. Marrow-derived stromal cells express genes encoding a broad spectrum of arteriogenic cytokines and promote in vitro and in vivo arteriogenesis through paracrine mechanisms. Cir Res 2004;94:678–85.

[61] Bernardo ME, Fibbe WE. Mesenchymal stromal cells: sensors and switchers of inflammation. Cell Stem Cell 2013;13:392–402.

[62] Prockop DJ, Oh JY. Mesenchymal stem/stromal cells (MSCs): role as guardians of inflammation. Mol Ther 2012;20:14–20.

[63] Timmermans F, De Sutter J, Gillebert TC. Stem cells for the heart, are we there yet? Cardiology 2003;100:176–85.

[64] Kinnaird T, Stabile E, Burnett MS, Epstein SE. Bone-marrow-derived cells for enhancing collateral development: mechanisms, animal data, and initial clinical experiences. Circ Res 2004;95:354–63.

[65] Murphy MP, et al. Autologous bone marrow mononuclear cell therapy is safe and promotes amputation-free survival in patients with critical limb ischemia. J Vasc Surg 2011;53:1565–74.

[66] Franz RW, et al. Use of autologous bone marrow mononuclear cell implantation therapy as a limb salvage procedure in patients with severe peripheral arterial disease. J Vasc Surg 2009;50:1378–90.

[67] Benoit E, et al. The role of amputation as an outcome measure in cellular therapy for critical limb ischemia: implications for clinical trial design. J Transl Med 2011;9:165.

[68] Teraa M, et al. Autologous bone marrow-derived cell therapy in patients with critical limb ischemia: a meta-analysis of randomized controlled clinical trials. Ann Surg 2013;258:922–9.

[69] Arai M, et al. Granulocyte colony-stimulating factor: a noninvasive regeneration therapy for treating atherosclerotic peripheral artery disease. Circ J 2006;70:1093–8.

[70] Matoba S, et al. Long-term clinical outcome after intramuscular implantation of bone marrow mononuclear cells (Therapeutic Angiogenesis by Cell Transplantation [TACT] trial) in patients with chronic limb ischemia. Am Heart J 2008;156:1010–8.

[71] Norgren L, et al. Inter-society consensus for the management of peripheral arterial disease (TASC II). J Vasc Surg 2007;45(Suppl S):S5–67.

[72] Klinkert P, van Dijk PJ, Breslau PJ. Polytetrafluoroethylene femorotibial bypass grafting: 5-year patency and limb salvage. Ann Vasc Surg 2003;17:486–91.

[73] Wen Y, Meng L, Gao Q. Autologous bone marrow cell therapy for patients with peripheral arterial disease: a meta-analysis of randomized controlled trials. Expert Opin Biol Ther 2011;11:1581–9.

[74] Huang P, et al. Autologous transplantation of granulocyte colony-stimulating factor-mobilized peripheral blood mononuclear cells improves critical limb ischemia in diabetes. Diabetes Care 2005;28:2155–60.

[75] Ozturk A, et al. Therapeutical potential of autologous peripheral blood mononuclear cell transplantation in patients with type 2 diabetic critical limb ischemia. J Diabetes Complications 2012;26:29–33.

[76] Mohammadzadeh L, et al. Therapeutic outcomes of transplanting autologous granulocyte colony-stimulating factor-mobilised peripheral mononuclear cells in diabetic patients with critical limb ischaemia. Exp Clin Endocrinol Diabetes 2013;121:48–53.

[77] Lu D, et al. Comparison of bone marrow mesenchymal stem cells with bone marrow-derived mononuclear cells for treatment of diabetic critical limb ischemia and foot ulcer: a double-blind, randomized, controlled trial. Diabetes Res Clin Pract 2011;92:26–36.

[78] Gupta PK, et al. A double blind randomized placebo controlled phase I/II study assessing the safety and efficacy of allogeneic bone marrow derived mesenchymal stem cell in critical limb ischemia. J Transl Med 2013;11:143.

[79] Fujita Y, et al. Phase II clinical trial of CD34+ cell therapy to explore endpoint selection and timing in patients with critical limb ischemia. Circulation 2014;78:490–501.

[80] Losordo DW, et al. A randomized, controlled pilot study of autologous CD34+ cell therapy for critical limb ischemia. Circulation 2012;5:821–30.

[81] Perin EC, et al. A randomized, controlled study of autologous therapy with bone marrow-derived aldehyde dehydrogenase bright cells in patients with critical limb ischemia. Catheter Cardiovasc Interv 2011;78:1060–7.

[82] Powell RJ, et al. Cellular therapy with Ixmyelocel-T to treat critical limb ischemia: the randomized, double-blind, placebo-controlled RESTORE-CLI trial. Mol Ther 2012;20:1280–6.

Chapter 4

Mesenchymal Stem Cells for Treatment of Peripheral Vascular Disease

T.J. Povsic, MD, PhD
Duke Clinical Research Institute, Duke Medicine, Durham, NC, United States

CLINICAL NEED

Peripheral vascular disease (PVD) is a highly prevalent disorder, estimated to affect 8–12 million Americans [1] and more than 25 million people in Europe and North America [2–4]. Although the development of PVD is associated with many of the same risk factors for coronary artery disease (CAD), patients with diabetes and those who smoke appear to be exceptionally susceptible to PVD.

The attention to PVD has significantly grown recently, influenced by the greater appreciation of the increased risk these patients have for morbidity and mortality [5], leading to greater emphasis on screening and detection of PVD in patients at risk for vascular disease and more aggressive therapy in patients found to have PVD. Indeed, several clinical trials are aimed at exploring the utility of more aggressive approaches to vascular disease treatment, specifically in patients with PVD.

PVD also leads to direct impairment in patients' quality and quantity of life via both of its predominant clinical manifestations: intermittent claudication (IC) and critical limb ischemia (CLI). Claudication impairs exercise capacity, limits mobility, and leads to increasing frailty and impairment in quality of life.

First-line therapy for patients with PVD includes risk factor modification, including smoking cessation. Revascularization is used to improve perfusion to the affected limb, ameliorate symptoms, and, in severe cases, affect limb salvage; however, at least in IC, the role of revascularization is under scrutiny. For instance, several studies suggest that exercise interventions are as, if not more, effective at improving exercise capacity and ameliorating symptoms in this condition. It is well established that exercise results in effective mobilization of a variety of stem cell types [6–9], suggesting that this intervention may represent

Regenerative Medicine for Peripheral Artery Disease. http://dx.doi.org/10.1016/B978-0-12-801344-1.00004-8

a type of "stem-cell" therapy for PVD. Smoking cessation may act similarly by removing a modifiable risk factor which leads to suppression of progenitor cell–mediated vascular reparative capacity [10].

A significant fraction of patients with PVD display progress of disease to CLI, in which obstruction of blood flow reaches a critical stage resulting in rest ischemic pain, ulcers, poor healing, susceptibility to infection, and ultimately threatened limb loss [4]. These patients display much higher morbidity and mortality of up to 20% per year [4]. Although revascularization remains at the forefront of attempts to affect wound healing and limb salvage in these patients, some studies estimate that up to 20–30% of patients with CLI are poor candidates for either surgical or endovascular revascularization [4,11]. Amputation for lower extremity PVD represents an extremely poor prognostic factor, with acute mortality of up to 30% and 5-year survival rates of less than 30% [12,13]. Estimates indicate that up to a quarter million amputations are performed in Europe and North America annually [14]; although, the results of a recent analysis suggest that rates of amputations are declining [15]. In addition to the risk of mortality, quality of life in these patients is similar to that of terminally ill patients with malignancies [16], and the health-care expenditure on these patients is estimated at almost $50,000 per patient per year [17]. Thus, the need for alternative therapies for these patients remains a paramount medical need.

How diseases such as PVD develop and how regenerative therapies might be used to improve outcomes is unclear. For instance, ischemic and injured tissue is constantly being perfused with circulating progenitor cells of various types, including cells capable of mesenchymal properties [18,19]. One theory of vascular injury and disease (Fig. 4.1) is that chronic vascular injury leads to an initial mobilization of stem cells [20–25]. Although initially capable of affecting repair and healing, chronic injury eventually leads to depletion of stem-cell capacity [26–29], at which point repair is no longer affected and clinically evident disease ensues [30–32].

The promise of stem-cell therapy is that by augmenting and supplementing native cell-mediated repair, perhaps via stimulation of local stem cells through paracrine signaling [33–35], efficient and thorough repair and greater healing will lead to an interruption of this cycle of ongoing injury followed by inadequate tissue restoration. By "boosting" repair, the administration of stem cells might reset this reparative mechanism to a point where capacity is adequate to maintain tissue integrity, allowing the organism to resist future injury, maintain physical functioning, and prevent overt disease.

MESENCHYMAL STEM CELLS

Mesenchymal stem cells (MSCs) fulfill many of the criteria for an ideal adult stem cell for regenerative therapy for a variety of conditions including PVD. Identified over 30 years ago [36], MSCs are derived from the

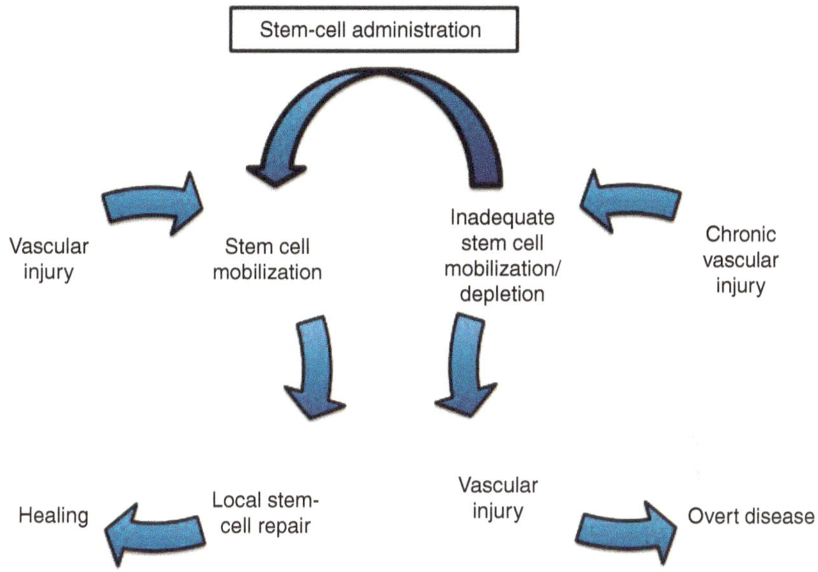

FIGURE 4.1 **Schematic of a model of chronic (vascular) injury and stem-cell-mediated repair.**

stromal fraction of bone marrow, and can be readily isolated and identified on the basis of growth and expansion on plastic surfaces. MSCs are easily grown and expanded from bone marrow [37], have multilineage potential [38–41], and appear to exhibit immunological tolerance [42]. Although easily isolated and expanded, MSCs are more difficult to characterize using conventional techniques, most notably, expression of unique and identifying cell-surface markers. One recent proposal from the International Society for Cell Therapy identified MSCs on the basis of their adherence of plastic surfaces; expression of cell surface CD73, CD90, and CD105; lack of expression of cell-surface expression of CD34, CD45, HLA-DR, CD14, CD79a, or CD19; and multilineage differentiation capacity [43]. Despite this attempt at standardization, it appears clear that MSCs isolated from differing tissues and/or under different conditions likely result in distinct stem or more differentiated but still multipotent progenitor cells, characterized by differences in gene expression. The biological consequences of these variations may be significant, and one should remain cognizant that MSCs across studies are unlikely to represent uniform or identical cell types [44,45]. Details regarding isolation and expansion techniques may result in significant clinical sequelae. Despite these limitations, MSCs remain of great clinical interest given the favorable properties previously discussed.

MESENCHYMAL STEM CELLS AND ANGIOGENESIS

A mouse hindlimb ischemia model was frequently, if not almost exclusively, used for the initial development of a variety of angiogenic and regenerative approaches to cardiovascular disease, dating to the original description of an endothelial progenitor cell by Asahara et al. [46], a seminal experiment that demonstrated that these cells could improve distal perfusion after femoral artery ligation. This model has demonstrated the utility of both unselected [47] and stromal bone marrow [48] cells on improving perfusion, likely via collateral vessel growth, establishing the possibility of using cell sources that contain either mixtures of cells including MSCs or selected MSCs for therapeutic angiogenesis.

Various mesenchymal cells have been studied in hindlimb ischemia models. Prather et al. demonstrated that administration of PLX-PAD cells, derived from human placental tissue, results in improvements in blood flow, capillary density, and reduced oxidative stress [49]. Cells selected for high aldehyde dehydrogenase activity ($ALDH^{br}$ of $ALDH^{bright}$ cells) represent another MSC-enriched population, although ALDH is a marker of a variety of stem-cell phenotypes including endothelial and hematopoietic progenitors [50–54]. In a hindlimb ischemia model, these cells were likewise able to significantly improve distal perfusion. Capoccia et al. demonstrated that purification of this population resulted in an enhanced stem-cell product with improved perfusion and increased capillary density in animals treated with purified $ALDH^{br}$ cells, even when the unpurified product contained greater numbers of unpurified $ALDH^{br}$ cells [55]. This mirrors the findings with $CD34^+$ cells and suggests that cell purification may be an important component to greater efficacy of regenerative products [56].

Interestingly, in these models, multiple researchers have suggested that mixtures of cells may be more efficacious than isolated endothelial cell populations. For instance, Asahara demonstrated that coculture of $CD34^+$ cells with non-CD34 expressing cells improved bioactivity compared with the use of "endothelial progenitor cells" (EPCs) ($CD34^+$ cells) alone [46]. Similar findings have been demonstrated in early clinical studies in which the use of unselected bone marrow populations were more efficacious than isolated hematopoietic stem cells [57,58]. In addition, studies in which bone marrow cells were compared with peripheral mononuclear cells (likely lacking the MSC component) have concluded that the interaction between CD34+ "EPCs" with cells lacking capability of directly incorporating into the vasculature but supplying key angiogenic paracrine factors was responsible for the greater efficacy of bone marrow cells observed [59]. These observations were not replicated when comparing bone marrow cells with circulating peripheral stem cells obtained after G-CSF mobilization [60]. Concluding whether this is due to partial mobilization of MSCs into the circulation by G-CSF or other differences between the trials and cell types would require additional head-to-head comparisons.

The hypothesis that multiple cell types may be required for maximal efficacy corroborates observations that mixed cell lines lead to more robust vascular (tubule) development in in vitro experiments [61–63], suggesting that multiple cell types work in concert to effect vasculogenesis.

COMPARISON OF ISOLATED MESENCHYMAL STEM CELLS WITH OTHER CELL POPULATIONS: PRECLINICAL STUDIES

Metaanalyses have suggested that administration of unselected bone marrow cells in the days following acute myocardial infarction leads to a small but significant improvement in ejection fraction [64–66], an effect that appears to translate into a clinically important impact on cardiovascular events [65,67]. Whether or not MSCs might prove to be more powerful effectors of tissue salvage and improve perfusion remains to be determined, however, several direct comparisons in animal models have suggested that MSCs may be more powerful effectors of myocardial repair.

In an acute myocardial infarction model, Li et al. compared the efficacy and potency of four stem cell types that were or are being evaluated clinically in a variety of cardiovascular indications, including several mesenchymal or mesenchymal-like populations as well as unselected bone marrow mononuclear cells [68]. In particular, cardiac derived cells (CDCs) were characterized as expressing high levels of CD105 (>99%) and low expression of CD90 (<18%), whereas bone marrow and adipose-derived-mesenchymal stem cells (Ad-MSCs) expressed both these markers to high levels (>99% and >85%, respectively). These authors characterized the secretion of a variety of proangiogenic and other growth factors felt to be important to cardiac recovery including angiopoietin-2 (Ang-2), basic fibroblast growth factor (bFGF), human growth factor (HGF), insulin-like growth factor-1 (IGF-1), stromal-derived factor-1 (SDF-1), and vascular endothelial growth factor (VEGF). Each of these was expressed at highest levels by cardiosphere-derived cells, whereas selected MSCs secreted higher levels of Ang-2, bFGF, SDF-1, and VEGF compared with unselected bone marrow cells. These cells were also markedly superior to bone marrow cells in in vitro tube formation, a marker of angiogenesis. In a postinfarct model, there was greater improvement in ejection fraction with each of the selected MSCs in comparison with unselected bone marrow cells [68].

In a porcine acute myocardial infarction model, infusion of late-outgrowth EPCs, MSCs, or control vehicle were compared. In contrast to previous studies, late outgrowth EPCs were shown to secrete higher levels of the proangiogenic growth factor placental growth factor, although MSCs secreted higher levels of VEGF, IGF-1, while late-outgrowth EPCs better incorporated into new blood vessels and demonstrated dramatic improvements in vascular density in the infarct zone; however, cardiac magnetic resonance imaging (MRI) assessments suggested the EPCs and MSCs were associated with similar decreases in infarct size, bringing into question whether or to what degree vascular density was associated with functional recovery [69].

In a permanent ligation acute MI model, Armiñán et al. compared human bone marrow MSCs with freshly isolated CD34+ cells from umbilical-cord blood [70]. Fractional shortening, fractional area change, and anterior wall thickening were all improved with both cell types; however, MSCs were associated with a numerically higher degree of anterior wall thickening, and statistically significant reductions in scar tissue compared with either CD34+ isolated cells or placebo treatment. In this model, the degree of vascular density was improved to a similar degree by both MSCs and $CD34^+$ cells.

Finally, in a rat hindlimb ischemia model, MSC administration was associated with higher level of improvements in regional blood flow, limb necrosis and self-amputation, and global hindlimb perfusion [71]. Interestingly, in this vascular bed, MSC therapy was associated with a higher level of vascular density compared with either control treatment or mononuclear cell (MNC) therapy. As in previous studies, these in vivo findings were associated with higher levels of secretion of proangiogenic growth factors, in this case VEGF, bFGF, and a markedly higher level of SDF-1 expression which was not detected in the mononuclear cells used in this study [71].

In summary, these studies suggest that MSCs may be particularly attractive populations of cells for the treatment of ischemic tissue, including underperfused peripheral vascular beds as well as critically ischemic limbs. The findings that similar results were obtained in ischemic brain tissue [72] may speak to a commonality of mechanisms inherent in the treatment of ischemic tissues regardless of organ, or to the plasticity of the MSC population, which given its pluripotential properties, may be particularly suited for treatment of a variety of ischemic substrates.

COMPARISON OF ISOLATED MESENCHYMAL STEM CELLS WITH OTHER CELL POPULATIONS: CLINICAL STUDIES

Small studies have compared MSCs with other cell sources in humans. In the TAC-HFT trial, Feldman and coworkers randomized 65 participants with ischemic cardiomyopathy to treatment with autologous MSCs or autologous unselected bone marrow cells. Because administration of these cells occurs at different time points after randomization, each patient underwent a serial randomization to treatment cell type, and then between cell therapy treatment and placebo [73]. Although the study is too small to be definitive, there are intriguing signals that MSC therapy might be more potent than the use of unselected marrow populations, as reflected in improvements in distance walked in 6 min, infarct size as measured using MRI, and regional recovery [74].

The utility of selected bone marrow cells was also demonstrated in an infarct model where cells expressing the hematopoietic and endothelial marker CD34 were compared with unselected marrow cells. Treatment with a cell product with purified cells resulted in greater myocardial recovery, higher levels of angiogenesis, and lower levels of fibrosis compared with an unselected cell product containing the same numbers of $CD34^+$ cells [56].

Whether these results are directly applicable to the treatment of PVD is unknown, however, given that the goal of this therapy is angiogenesis, similar to the goal in treatment of myocardial ischemia, it is reasonable to consider that similar results might be observed. A single study [75] comparing MSCs versus MNCs for the treatment of chronic limb ischemia demonstrated results consistent with those of Li et al. [68], demonstrating markedly higher levels of VEGF, FGF-2, and Ang-2 expression in cultured medium of either normally or hypoxic MSCs compared with bone marrow MNCs. Patients were randomized to therapy with either MSCs or bone marrow MNCs, then further randomized to cell injection or placebo. Although patients treated with either cell type improved, there were some differences noted between the two treatment strategies: notably, there was no difference in improvement in rest pain between the groups, however, pain-free walking time improved to a greater extent in the MSC group, as did improvements in ankle–brachial index (ABI), and $TcPO_2$. Analysis using magnetic resonance angiography demonstrated improvements in the numbers of collateral vessels in MSC-treated patients compared with either MNC- or control-treated patients. Remarkably, the number of healing ulcers in the MSC group was significantly higher than the control injection group, and ulcer healing was also improved and occurred earlier than noted in the MNC group [75]

CLINICAL TRIALS DESIGN CONSIDERATIONS

The development of regenerative therapies for treatment of PVD has been of significant clinical interest since the first cell therapies were being developed for cardiovascular disease. Indeed, early meetings in the field generated significant debate about the relative ease of trials in PVD versus other cardiovascular indications. These debates continue to frame the challenges and opportunities in the field.

The dual manifestations of PVD, IC, and CLI represent essentially disparate disease states dictating divergent biological considerations and trial designs. Why some patients develop and present with CLI, whereas others with severe PVD manifest only IC, remains unknown; however, some studies suggest that underlying differences in biology or genetics may be the basis of these differential expressions of vascular disease. Whether these biological differences should impact clinical development programs remains largely unknown but of theoretical concern. For instance, CLI may represent more "end-stage" disease, in which autologous cell sources are either further depleted or functionally impaired, findings which may impact the utility of autologous cell sources unless they can be artificially manipulated and regenerated.

Unique to PVD is relatively easy access to the affected tissue, which has implications both for ease and safety of administration of the cell product as well as easier justification of a "double-blind" trial design in which all patients undergo administration of study product in a fully blinded design. Such considerations are especially vital when subjective endpoints such as wound healing and walking distance represent trial endpoints. In addition, the relative ease of peripheral biopsy has implications for the possibility of mechanistic analysis before and after therapy.

TREATMENT OF CRITICAL LIMB ISCHEMIA

Critical limb ischemia is the more studied manifestation of PVD. Factors that have led investigators to target this disease include: (1) the immense clinical need, as reflected by the very high morbidity and mortality in these patients with estimates of up to a 20% mortality rate per year [76,77]; and (2) the lack of other therapies for these patients, and (in theory) the presence of a "hard" clinical endpoint (amputation) which, if curtailed, would lead to a direct pathway to clinical approval and reimbursement. Indeed, the clinical need is reflected in the immense health-care costs associated with treatment of these subjects, which has been estimated to exceed $47,000 per year.

Unfortunately, the execution of these trials has proven difficult due to several concerns that impact clinical trial design: (1) there is large regional variability in the use of amputation [15], an effect that is likely exacerbated when one considers international studies where differences in the approach to amputation make prediction of rates of outcomes difficult; (2) differences in willingness to proceed with amputation on the basis of known or perceived treatment assignment may place inherent biases in the trial; (3) the possibility that amputation rates in general may be decreasing will make completion of adequately powered studies more difficult [15]; (4) concerns about off-target effects and potential exacerbation of diabetic retinopathy in particular make enrollment criteria restrictive, given that patients with this most advanced manifestation of PVD typically have an extremely high burden of comorbidities and are frequently characterized by advanced diabetes; (5) this high burden of comorbid conditions makes the incidence of adverse events high; and (6) the rate of amputation is highly variable between different manifestations of CLI, with rates of amputation extremely high in patients with readily apparent tissue loss, but much lower in patients whose only clinical manifestation of CLI is rest pain. Finally, there is a theoretical concern that in patients with tissue loss, the extent of injury is so highly advanced that the opportunity for repair has been lost. This may be especially applicable to cell therapies, in which there are preclinical and clinical data that cell products obtained from older patients with higher levels of comorbidities or more advanced ischemic disease [78] may lack reparative capacity, an underlying hypothesis of the "repair exhaustion" theory for the development of vascular disease [18,28–31].

The difficulty of clinical investigation in this field is highlighted by the experience in the development of FGF in this context. Although a phase-II study

(TALISMAN, NCT 00798005) reported a significant improvement in amputation-free survival in the 125 randomized patients (73% in FGF-treated patients compared with 52% in control patients) [79], these results were associated with an improvement in mortality (12% vs 23%), and the combined endpoint of major amputations and death was significantly reduced (HR = 0.44, $p = 0.01$). These exciting results led to the execution of a phase-III trial (TAMARIS), the results of which were highly anticipated given the size of the study ($n = 525$ from over 30 countries), but disappointing in that amputation rates were virtually identical in the two groups (36% [FGF] vs 33% [placebo]) [80], mirroring what was observed in the control group of the phase-II study.

One key advantage of investigating CLI is the opportunity to obtain pathological analysis of tissue removed at the time of any future amputation. Although the amount of data in this regard is limited, at least one study noted the presence of neovasculature in the area of cell injection, an observation not made in a control population [81]. Similar mechanistic substudies were performed as part of the TALISMAN investigation, verifying local gene expression [82].

UNSELECTED MESENCHYMAL STEM CELL POPULATIONS

Many trials have investigated the use of minimally manipulated cell populations containing MSCs for treatment of CLI (Table 4.1). The studies have usually targeted Rutherford class 4–6 patients with atherosclerotic disease, although some have included patients with Beurger's disease and vasculitides. The majority of these trials were small, nonrandomized feasibility studies exploring the use of a variety of cell isolation and selection techniques or seeking biological signals of cell activity [86–98]. Although many early phase, uncontrolled, nonrandomized studies have been reported, the focus here will be on studies in which a meaningful comparison with a control population is available (Table 4.1).

The therapeutic angiogenesis using cell transplantation study (TACT) likely represents the largest single experience in this arena, and compared unselected bone marrow cells with cells from the peripheral circulation in patients with bilateral ischemia in which both legs were injected [59]. This study encompassed several phases. In the pilot phase, 25 patients with unilateral ischemia were studied. In this phase, there was virtually no change in ABI, $TcPO_2$, rest pain, or new collateral formation in the patients treated with saline, while ABI improved by 0.13, $TcPO_2$ by 19 mmHg, and rest pain by −2.6 units at 4 weeks. At 24 weeks, the values were almost identical to those observed at 4 weeks. Differences between the treated and control groups for each of these parameters was highly statistically significant ($p < 0.0001$ for all assessments).

This was followed by a second "B" phase, which enrolled 22 patients with bilateral ischemia randomized to treatment with bone marrow MNCs in one side and peripheral blood MNCs on the other. Treatment with bone marrow cells resulted in improvements in both ABI (difference between groups of 0.09, $p < 0.0001$) and $TcPO_2$ (difference between groups of 13 mmHg, $p < 0.0001$)

TABLE 4.1 Selected Randomized Controlled Studies of Unselected Cells for PVD

Study	Year	*N*	Population	Follow-up	Control	Design	Txt	Outcomes					
								A	$TcPO_2$	ABI	UH	WD	Pain
TACT-phase A [59]	2002	25	R4-6	24 weeks	None	Open	IM		+	+			+
TACT-phase B [59]	2002	22	R4-6	24 weeks	Placebo in other leg	R, B	IM		+	+	+	+	+
PROVASA [83]	2011	40	R4-6	3 months	Placebo	R, DB	IA	–		+	+		
TAM-PAD [84]	2007	13	R3-6	13 months	Matched	R	IA + IM			+		+	
Huang et al. [60]	2007	150	R4-6		PB MNCs versus BM MNCs	R, DB	IM	–	–	+	–	–	+
ACT-34 CLI [85]	2012	28	R4-5	1 year	CD34+ cells	R, DB	IM	+			+	–	+

Population: *R*, Rutherford class;
Study design: *R*, randomized; *DB*, double blind;
Delivery: *IA*, intraarterial; *IM*, intramuscular;
Outcomes: *A*, amputation; *ABI*, ankle brachial index; *TcPO*$_{2P}$, transcutaneous oximetry; *UH*, ulcer healing; *WD*, walking distance; +, outcome improved; –, no effect.

compared with cells peripheral blood MNCs, which typically lack MSC populations. Perhaps most remarkably, rest pain resolved in 16 of 20 bone marrow cell-treated patients versus only 3 of 20 patients treated with peripheral blood cells. These results remained robust at 24-week follow-up. Notably, the changes in each parameter between patients treated with bone marrow cells in groups A and B were remarkably consistent, while the effect of peripheral blood MNCs appeared modest at best, with essentially no change in ABI and markedly smaller effects on $TcPO_2$ and rest pain compared with bone marrow cells.

The group also published a study that included up to 3 years of follow-up. This study included 115 patients, 74 with peripheral arterial disease (PAD) and 41 with thromboangiitis obliterans (TAO) [99], due to an expansion of enrollment from the initial three hospitals in the TACT study [59] to 10 in this follow-up report. It appears that further patients were not randomized but were treated with open-label bone-marrow cell product. It is not possible to draw any firm conclusions about efficacy, but a few observations from this study are of interest: (1) the demographics, outcomes, and amputation rates from the PAD and TAO populations were significantly different, reflecting the differences between these disease states; (2) in patients with PAD, the vast majority (83%) of amputations occurred within 6 months of cell therapy, the time period during which comparisons between the treated and control patients were available in the initial TACT report [59], suggesting that if cell therapy is to have an impact on this important endpoint, an effect may be observed relatively quickly; (3) evaluation of other endpoints of tissue perfusion such as ABI and $TcPO_2$ showed much more modest effects than were observed in the initial report [59], again cautioning against overinterpretation of data from small studies; and (4) perhaps expectedly, the majority of changes in other clinical markers (rest pain, claudication distance, ulcer size) were observed within the first 6 months.

This last observation points to a key unresolved issue in cell therapy trials, which is the need or requirement for multiple dosing strategies. To date, there are almost no data on treating patients with multiple doses of cells. Although it is conceivable that a single treatment might reverse a cycle in which tissue destruction (Fig. 4.1) leading to impairment in ability to walk and mobilize additional reparative circulating stem cells results in a progressive cycle of additional damage, it is rare for a single treatment of any therapy to have such a profound effect.

These investigators took advantage of the possibilities for tissue retrieval when treating substrates likely to require amputation or excision, demonstrating neovascularization distal to sites of injection [100].

The PROVASA study randomized 40 patients to intraarterial cell therapy versus placebo [83]. Although cell therapy resulted in intriguing benefits in ABI, the trial was limited as only 3 months of analysis were completed before crossover was allowed, severely limiting the conclusions that could be drawn especially since many trials have suggested that the effects of cell therapy may be more prominent in the 6–12 month time frame [101].

COMPARISON OF MESENCHYMAL STEM CELLS WITH OTHER CELL TYPES

Several trials have compared cell types. Conclusions from these studies need to be limited: (1) there is likely to be a significant placebo effect in all patients, since in almost all cases, no control group is included; and (2) a staple of the evaluation of new therapeutics should be that effect sizes for most interventions are almost always modest, thus studies that compare interventions are, by nature, exceedingly difficult since they require comparison of two interventions, and one can expect the difference in effect between the two arms to be even smaller than what would be observed in a placebo-controlled study. The TACT trial largely found that treatment with peripheral blood MNCs was ineffective, mirroring what was found in the placebo group from the initial pilot study; thus, the power of this study was improved due to lack of efficacy in one of the interventions [59]. Numerically, however, it appears that some of the dramatic benefits observed initially were less impressive in a follow-up uncontrolled study, in which no improvement in ABI was observed [99].

A larger study of stem-cell therapy for the treatment of lower-limb arteriosclerosis obliterans built on early work assessing the treatment of this disease by a group in China [102,103]. This group randomized 150 patients to treatment with multiple doses of either stem cells obtained after mobilization with granulocyte colony stimulating factor (G-CSF) or from bone marrow aspiration [104]. Notably, the numbers of cells that were implanted in the peripheral blood group appear to be about 10× higher than that obtained from bone marrow aspiration; however, improvements in all parameters were significantly better in the patients treated with bone marrow cells including improvement in rest pain and pain-free walking distance. Although there was some suggestion that the opposite was true for effect on ABI, it is notable that the baseline ABI in the patients receiving peripheral blood treatment was lower (0.47 vs 0.53, $p = 0.06$), and the final ABI in both groups was 0.63.

Although not directly assessing the role of MSCs, an important contribution to the literature in this field is the study of mobilized stem cells enriched in an endothelial phenotype, perhaps the most rigorously performed trial in this area, representing a completely double-blinded, placebo-controlled design. In this study [105], 28 patients were randomized to either low $-(1 \times 10^5)$ or high-dose (1×10^6) autologous $CD34^+$ cells, or placebo. Remarkably, in this completely blinded study, there was a difference in amputation rates between the groups, with 67% of control subjects, 43% of low-dose subjects, and only 22% of high-dose cell-treated subjects experiencing this endpoint at 6 months. Comparison of the 12-month rates of amputation in the cell therapy groups (31.3%) with control patients (75%) was nominally statistically significant ($p = 0.05$).

Although these data should not be overinterpreted, they do suggest that some of the efficacy observed in other studies may stand up in the face of a double-blind design, in which clinical decision making is not influenced by knowledge of treatment assignment, a severe limitation of other trial designs.

MESENCHYMAL STEM CELLS FOR INTERMITTENT CLAUDICATION

The TAM-PAD study represents the only clinical trial that appears to have exclusively included patients with IC (Rutherford class 3 CLI), and compared intraarterial and intramuscular cell therapy with a matched but nonrandomized control group. This study incorporated a number of small modifications that assessed unique aspects of cell therapy, although given the number of patients enrolled, the conclusions that can be drawn are limited [84].

In this controlled, but open-label study, 13 patients underwent both intraarterial and intramuscular treatment with cell product. In addition, prior to cell therapy, the peripheral tissue bed was made ischemic by having patients exercise on bicycles until they felt ischemic pain, and inducing further ischemia using a blood pressure cuff to exceed systemic systolic blood pressure, thereby creating an ischemic signal to stimulate stem-cell homing and retention.

The patients treated with stem-cell therapy had a remarkable 3.5-fold increase in their walking distance from 147 to 500 m (2 months) and subsequently to 542 m (13 months). In contrast, the open-label controls had no change in exercise time. Other measures of perfusion were also improved at 2 months, including venous oxygen saturation (59–56%, $p = 0.005$), peak blood flow (2.1–2.5, $p = 0.09$), and averaged reactive hyperemia (5.3–7.2, $p = 0.003$). Peak blood flow also rose from 5.3 to 7.2 ($p = 0003$). These values were largely maintained at 13 months, although the actual data for these findings are not presented in the manuscript.

It should be noted that the control subjects were not eligible for stem-cell therapy due to concurrent coronary disease or other contraindications to trial participation, factors that could influence stem-cell biology and potency as well as which might impact the patients' motivation to exercise and improve their clinical condition, impacting the comparison are presented here.

Although the findings were suggestive, including improvements in ABI, capillary oxygen saturation, and pain-free walking distance, the nonrandomized design and possibility of a significant placebo effect in this open-label design merits caution in interpretation [84].

METAANALYSIS

To date, a single metaanalysis of all stem-cell-related trials for PVD has attempted to assess the impact of cell therapy on both surrogate markers of ischemia, symptoms, and hard endpoints of ulcer healing and amputation [105]. Over a short range of follow-up (median follow-up 6 months), this analysis suggested a favorable and highly statistically significant impact on ABI from 0.46

to 0.64 ($p = 0.011$). $TcPO_2$ increased from 22.8 to 35.8 ($p = 0.0002$), and walking distance increased from 75.7 to 402.3 m ($p < 0.001$). The rate of amputation was assessed in only two trials, one randomized [102] and one nonrandomized [106], yielding on odds ratio of 0.09 (CI 0.02 – 0.44, $p = 0.0005$). In addition, this study predates more recent studies, including the data from Losordo et al., which showed significant trends toward lower amputation rates in cell-treated subjects [85].

Of note, the impact when assessing only controlled clinical trials was dramatically decreased, and in most cases, no longer statistically significant. This points to the immense need for adequately placebo-controlled, randomized, and blinded studies. Unfortunately, in this field, even the majority of placebo-controlled trials were open-label, and may be subject to significant bias.

ISOLATED MESENCHYMAL STEM CELLS

There has been limited study of purified MSCs for the treatment of PVD, although their pluripotent potential and antiinflammatory properties may make them ideal in this regard. Indeed, MSCs are being studied in a variety of conditions, including sepsis and other inflammatory states, which also suggest that these cells may be particularly attractive to conditions associated with severe PVD, including limited wound healing. Nonetheless, several studies of stem-cell products, which are at minimum enriched for MSCs, have been completed or are ongoing (Tables 4.2 and 4.3).

Two concurrent phase-I trials of placental-derived stem cells for the treatment of CLI have been completed and presented. These trials enrolled a total of 27 patients in a European and US study in variable dosing cohorts to determine tolerability and safety, as well as to assess for potential sensitization via immunological responses in these patients. A subset of patients received repeat dosing separated by a 2-week interval. A comprehensive immunological evaluation demonstrated no concerns, and adverse events were comparable with the placebo-treated patients. The majority of subjects reported improvements in quality of life and pain scores, but the size of these studies precludes any efficacy assessments. Currently, a phase-II trial is recruiting patients in IC, and Pluristem Therapeutics Inc. (Haifa, Israel) has pursued expansion of this study with enrollment in Korea, Germany, Israel, and the United States. The sponsor is pursuing early approval of PLX-PAD through the new adaptive pathways pilot project of the European Medicines Agency as well as the Accelerated Pathway for Regenerative Medicine in Japan.

Ixmyelocel-T is an autologous product being developed by Aastrom Inc. (now Vericel Corporation), which is obtained via a culture process of bone-marrow-harvested product [107]. Similar to $ALDH^{br}$ cells, Ix cells likely represent not only a mixture of cell types including hematopoietic cells but also MSCs that express CD90, as the number of cells expressing this marker is highly enriched during the culturing process and in the final Ix product. A phase-II

TABLE 4.2 Ongoing or Completed Studies of Isolated Mesenchymal Stem Cell Populations

NCT number	Sponsor	N	Phase	Cell	Cell type	Notes
NCT00392509	Aldagen	20	I/II	Selected on the basis of ALDH activity	BM cells selected for high ALDH activity, present in multiple stem cell types, including MSCs	I/II completed, II/III study not started Company acquired
NCT00523731	TheraVitae Ltd	6	I	Vescell	Autologous BM-cultured product	Provides open-label stem cell treatments in Thailand
NCT00951210	Pluristem Ltd	12	I	PLX-PAD	Placental-derived stem cell with multipotent properties, and high expression of MSC markers	
NCT00919958	Pluristem Ltd	15	I	PLX-PAD	Placental-derived stem cell with multipotent properties, and high expression of MSC markers	
NCT01472289	Cesca Therapeutics	15	I		Totipotent stem cell isolated from BM or UCB	Trial not enrolling, last updated Sep 2013
NCT01245335	Harves Technologies	210	II	Isolated MNCs		Currently not enrolling, enrollment not clear, website not updated
NCT01483898	Vericel	41	III			Not recruiting, no update since 2013
NCT00883870	Stempeutics Research Pvt Ltd	20	I, II	Allogenel MSCs	Allogenic MSCs from healthy donors	Unique allogenic therapy

ALDH, aldehyde dehydrogenase; *BM*, bone marrow; *MNC*, mononuclear cell; *MSC*, mesenchymal stem cell; *NCT*, national clinical trial; *UCB*, umbilical cord blood.

TABLE 4.3 Recruiting Studies of MSC Therapy for PVD

NCT number	Cell	Sponsor	Phase	N	Last updated	Primary completion date	Outcome measures
NCT01456819	MSCs	National University of Malaysia/ Cytopeutics Sdn Bhd	II	50	Apr. 2015	Dec. 2015	Change in angiogenesis, change in ulcer size, visual analog score, exercise treadmill test, improvement in vascularity and blood supply
NCT02099500	Auto adipose MSC	Ageless Regenerative Institute	I/II	200	Jul. 2014	Apr. 2016	ABI, collateral number, resolution of ulcer or gangrene, limb salvage
NCT01484574	Allogenic MSCs	Stempeutics Research Pvt Ltd	II	126	Feb. 2012	Sep. 2013	Relief of rest pain, healing of ulcerations or reduction of ulcer area, pain-free walking distance, major amputation-free survival, ABI, $TcPO_2$, QOL, collateral blood vessels by MRA
NCT01867190	ASCT01: Autologous stem cells	Lifecells, LLC	I/II	24	Sep. 2014	Dec. 2014	Major amputation (above the ankle) or persisting CLI (no clinical or perfusion improvement)
NCT02454231	CD14 + , CD34+ cells	University of Florence/Tuscany Region	II/III	38	May 2015	May 2015	$TcPO_2$, ABI, leg perfusion, QOL, amputation-free survival, improvement of microvascular anatomy
NCT00488020	Stem cells	Instituto de Molestias Cardiovasculares	I	10	Jun. 2008		Suppress pain and heal ischemic ulcers/ improve QOL
NCT02145897	Stromal fraction	Kasiak Research Pvt Ltd	I/II	60	May 2014	Aug. 2015	
NCT02336646	Allogenic MSCs	Taiwan Bio Therapeutics Co, Ltd	I	18	Jan. 2015	Aug. 2016	Relief of rest pain, perfusion as measured by ABI or $TcPO_2$, total walking distance on a standardized treadmill test

ABI, ankle brachial index; *CLI*, critical limb ischemia; *MSC*, mesenchymal stem cell; *NCT*, national clinical trial; *QOL*, quality of life.

study (RESTORE-CLI) enrolled 77 patients, of which 53 received therapy with Ix product whereas the rest were randomized to control treatment [108]. The study showed no safety concerns, with a statistically significant difference in the time to treatment failure, defined as all-cause mortality, major amputation of the index limb, or a doubling of the wound surface area from baseline. All components of the composite endpoint trended in a positive direction in cell-treated patients. Unfortunately, a phase-II study, reportedly being run under an agreed upon special protocol assessment with the US Food and Drug Administration (FDA), was stopped due to financial concerns and slow enrollment.

Aldehyde dehydrogenase can be used to isolate pluripotent cells enriched for MSCs and other stem cells [52]. They were studied in a proof-of-concept study using administration of unselected bone marrow cells as a control group [109]. Patients treated with $ALDH^{br}$ cells showed significant improvements in Rutherford category from baseline to 12 weeks. ABIs were also improved at both 6 and 12 weeks compared with baseline whereas patients treated with bone marrow MNCs showed no significant improvements at 6 or 12 weeks in Rutherford category, although they did show similar improvements in ABI. Neither therapy resulted in a significant change in $TcPO_2$ nor ischemic ulcer grade. A later phase trial was planned, but never consummated. Aldagen Inc., has since been acquired by Cytomedix., now Nuo Therapeutics. $ALDH^{br}$ cells are currently being evaluated in the National Institutes of Health-sponsored CCTRN run PACE (Clinical and MR Imaging Assessments in Patients with Intermittent Claudication Following Injection of Bone Marrow Derived ALDH Bright Cells) trial [110]. Other previously planned trials included a trial sponsored by Medistem Inc. (San Diego, CA), evaluating endometrial MSCs; however, as of this writing, this trial has also not commenced and its status is listed as unknown on ClinicalTrials.org [111].

A variety of other approaches are being tested in early phase clinical studies [3]. As shown, most of these studies are sponsored by foreign academic/hospital institutions, and over half have not been updated in over a year, suggesting that the status of enrollment and the studies are not clearly known. Additional planned studies (Table 4.4) indicate novel approaches, including the use of umbilical-cord blood cells and endometrial MSCs; however, the lack of recent updates is concerning and may indicate lack of sponsor funding or difficulties in enrollment.

REMAINING CHALLENGES

As with most other human clinical conditions, animal models in which to test new therapies are severely deficient. The hindlimb ischemia model has been used for years to assess for antiischemic properties of various cell therapies and has demonstrated that circulating cells both hone to and incorporate into new vasculature [46,112,113]. However, as with most animal models, the injury is acute and in an otherwise healthy animal. This hardly reflects the

degenerative, inflammatory, and chronic degenerative processes that characterize human disease.

A critical difficulty in the study of treatment of PVD is the lack of surrogate endpoints that might be used to reliably predict harder clinical endpoints; to date, these surrogate endpoints have not been accepted by regulatory agencies for the approval of novel therapies for this indication; the FDA in particular has remained committed to an endpoint of death and amputation free survival as the requirements for approval. Although ABI and $TcPO_2$ are associated with prognosis in population studies, it is not clear what the clinical impact of changes in these parameters mean in the context of improvements after therapy.

One possible solution to this conundrum is the use of patient-centered outcomes to assess the overall impact of the therapy in the clinic. In this regard, given the tight association of exercise time with clinical outcomes [114,115], outcomes such as walking distance might be of particular interest and value. In a different clinical context, this has been accepted by the FDA as an approvable endpoint when assessed in a placebo-controlled, double-blind design [116]. Alternatively, other investigators have explored the use of a series of patient-centered endpoints in a hierarchical design to assess the impact of the therapy on all aspects of patient care. This design has been used in other trials and has been proposed as a more powerful methodology for assessing clinical effects [117–119].

Alternatively, imaging capable of assessing microvascular perfusion would be of particular benefit to this field [120–124]. Although a wide variety of modalities have been explored, perhaps the use of MRI appears most promising. Of interest is the acceptance of this as a surrogate marker in the currently enrolling PACE trial being run by the NIH-sponsored Cell Therapy Clinical Trials Network (CCTRN). The PACET trial is assessing the utility of $ALDH^{br}$ cells, an enriched MSC population, for treatment of IC at eight US-based centers (NCT01774097) [110]. In this study, MRI will be used to assess leg collateral anatomy in addition to vascular flow using phase contrast magnetic resonance angiography to assess peak flow over time and perfusion using perfusion MRI, in which ischemia will be induced and the change in hyperemic fractional microvascular blood plasma volume over time will be assessed.

CONCLUSIONS

Experiences with the use of cell therapy for the treatment of PVD mirrors experiences with regenerative therapies for other cardiovascular conditions. There are many small feasibility studies that have not shown any significant safety concerns. Isolated MSCs, or stem cell populations which are enriched for MSCs, may be particularly potent in preclinical models, and some human experience supports the hypothesis that multiple stem cell types may be optimal. Although unselected bone marrow or purified populations have shown some promise, there are limited financial incentives for further development of these products. There are currently limited products in clinical trials. In particular, the recent experiences in cell-therapy trials, including cancellation of multiple studies in CLI, speak to the need for novel approaches in this field and engagement with regulatory authorities on new pathways to approval of these needed new treatments for patients with limited options.

REFERENCES

[1] Hirsch AT, Criqui MH, Treat-Jacobson D, et al. Peripheral arterial disease detection, awareness, and treatment in primary care. JAMA 2001;286(11):1317–24.

[2] Belch JF, Topol EJ, Agnelli G, et al. Critical issues in peripheral arterial disease detection and management: a call to action. Arch Int Med 2003;163(8):884–92.

[3] McDermott MMMD, Kerwin DRMD, Liu KP, Martin GJMD, O'Brien EBA, Kaplan HBA, et al. Prevalence and significance of unrecognized lower extremity peripheral arterial disease in general medicine practice. J Gen Int Med 2001;16(6):384–90.

[4] Norgren L, Hiatt WR, Dormandy JA, Nehler MR, Harris KA, Fowkes FGR. Inter-society consensus for the management of peripheral arterial disease (TASC II). J Vasc Surg 2007;45(1 Supplement):S5–S67.

[5] Ness J, Aronow WS. Prevalence of coexitence of coronary artery disease, ischemic stroke, and peripheral arterial disease in older persons, mean age 80 years, in an academic hospital based geriatrics practice. J Am Geriatr Soc 1999;47:1255.

[6] Fiorito C, Balestrieri ML, Crimi E, Giovane A, Grimaldi V, Minucci PB, et al. Effect of l-arginine on circulating endothelial progenitor cells and VEGF after moderate physical training in mice. Int J Cardiol 2008;126(3):421–3.

[7] Rehman J, Li J, Parvathaneni L, Karlsson G, Panchal VR, Temm CJ, et al. Exercise acutely increases circulating endothelial progenitor cells and monocyte-/macrophage-derived angiogenic cells. J Am Coll Cardiol 2004;43(12):2314–8.

[8] Sandri M, Adams V, Gielen S, Linke A, Lenk K, Krankel N, et al. Effects of exercise and ischemia on mobilization and functional activation of blood-derived progenitor cells in patients with ischemic syndromes: results of 3 randomized studies. Circulation 2005; 111(25):3391–9.

[9] Sarto P, Balducci E, Balconi G, Fiordaliso F, Merlo L, Tuzzato G, et al. Effects of exercise training on endothelial progenitor cells in patients with chronic heart failure. J Card Fail 2007;13(9):701–8.

[10] Kondo T, Hayashi M, Takeshita K, Numaguchi Y, Kobayashi K, Iino S, et al. Smoking cessation rapidly increases circulating progenitor cells in peripheral blood in chronic smokers. Arterioscler Thromb Vasc Biol 2004;24(8):1442–7.

[11] Lawall H, Bramlage P, Amann B. Treatment of peripheral arterial disease using stem and progenitor cell therapy. J Vasc Surg 2011;53(2):445–53.

[12] Adam DJ, Beard JD, Cleveland T, Bell J, Bradbury AW, Forbes JF, Fowkes FG, Gillepsie I, Ruckley CV, Raab G, Storkey H; BASIL trial participants. Bypass versus angioplasty in severe ischaemia of the leg (BASIL): multicentre, randomised controlled trial. Lancet 2005; 366(9501):1925–1934.

[13] Hirsch AT, Haskal ZJ, Hertzer NR, Bakal CW, Creager MA, Halperin JL, et al. ACC/AHA 2005 Practice Guidelines for the Management of Patients With Peripheral Arterial Disease (Lower Extremity, Renal, Mesenteric, and Abdominal Aortic): A collaborative report from

the American Association for Vascular Surgery/Society for Vascular Surgery,* Society for Cardiovascular Angiography and Interventions, Society for Vascular Medicine and Biology, Society of Interventional Radiology, and the ACC/AHA Task Force on Practice Guidelines (Writing Committee to Develop Guidelines for the Management of Patients With Peripheral Arterial Disease): Endorsed by the American Association of Cardiovascular and Pulmonary Rehabilitation; National Heart, Lung, and Blood Institute; Society for Vascular Nursing; TransAtlantic Inter-Society Consensus; and Vascular Disease Foundation. Circulation 2006;113(11):e463–654.

[14] Lawall H, Bramlage P, Amann B. Stem cell and progenitor cell therapy in peripheral artery disease: a critical appraisal. Thomb Haemost 2010;103:696–708.

[15] Jones WS, Patel MR, Dai D, Subherwal S, Stafford J, Calhoun S, Peterson ED. Temporal trends and geographic variation of lower-extremity amputation in patients with peripheral artery disease: results from U.S. Medicare 2000–2008. J Am Coll Cardiol 2012;60:2230–6.

[16] Albers M, Fratezi A, De Luccia N. Assissment of quality of life of patients with severe ischemia as a result of infrainguinal arterial occlusive disease. J Vasc Surg 1992;16:54–9.

[17] Eneroth M, Apelqvist J, Troeng T, Persson B. Operations, total hospital stay and costs of critical leg ischemia: a population-based, longitudinal outcome study of 321 patients. Acta Orthop Scand. 1996;67:459–65.

[18] Povsic T, Peterson ED. Stem cells for the ischaemic heart. Expert Opin Biol Ther 2006;6(5):427–42.

[19] Povsic T, Zavodni K, Kelly F, Zhu S, Goldschmidt-Clermont P, Dong C, et al. Circulating endogenous progenitor cells can be reliably identified on the basis of aldehyde dehydrogenase activity. J Am Coll Card 2007;53(20):2243–8.

[20] Leone AM, Rutella S, Bonanno G, Abbate A, Rebuzzi AG, Giovannini S, et al. Mobilization of bone marrow-derived stem cells after myocardial infarction and left ventricular function. Eur Heart J 2005;26(12):1196–204.

[21] Massa M, Rosti V, Ferrario M, Campanelli R, Ramajoli I, Rosso R, et al. Increased circulating hematopoietic and endothelial progenitor cells in the early phase of acute myocardial infarction. Blood 2005;105(1):199–206.

[22] Roberts N, Xiao Q, Weir G, Xu Q, Jahangiri M. Endothelial progenitor cells are mobilized after cardiac surgery. Ann Thorac Surg 2007;83(2):598–605.

[23] Shintani S, Murohara T, Ikeda H, Ueno T, Honma T, Katoh A, et al. Mobilization of endothelial progenitor cells in patients with acute myocardial infarction. Circulation 2001; 103:2776–9.

[24] Wojakowski W, Tendera M, Kucia M, Zuba-Surma E, Paczkowska E, Ciosek J, et al. Mobilization of bone marrow-derived Oct-4+ SSEA-4+ very small embryonic-like stem cells in patients with acute myocardial infarction. J Am Coll Cardiol 2009;53(1):1–9.

[25] Wojakowski W, Tendera M, Michalowska A, Majka M, Kucia M, Maslankiewicz K, et al. Mobilization of CD34/CXCR4+, CD34/CD117+, c-met+ stem cells, and mononuclear cells expressing early cardiac, muscle, and endothelial markers into peripheral blood in patients with acute myocardial infarction. Circulation 2004;110(20):3213–20.

[26] Inrig J, Van Buren P, Kim C, Vongpatanasin W, Povsic TJ, Toto R. Intradialytic hypertension is associated with endothelial cell dysfunction: results of the Mechanisms and Treatment of Intradialytic Hypertension (MATCH) Study. Clin J Am Soc Nephrol 2011;6(8):2016–24.

[27] Povsic TJ, Sloane R, Green JB, Zhou J, Pieper CF, Pearson MP, et al. Depletion of circulating progenitor cells precedes overt diabetes: a substudy from the VA enhanced fitness trial. J Diabetes Complications 2013;27(6):633–6.

[28] Povsic TJ, Sloane R, Zhou J, Pieper CF, Pearson MP, Peterson ED, et al. Lower levels of circulating progenitor cells are associated with low physical function and performance in elderly men with impaired glucose tolerance: a pilot substudy from the VA enhanced fitness trial. J Gerontol Ser A 2013;68(12):1559–66.
[29] Povsic TJ, Zhou J, Adams SD, Bolognesi MP, Attarian DE, Peterson ED. Aging is not associated with bone marrow-resident progenitor cell depletion. J Gerontol Ser A 2010;65A(10):1042–50.
[30] Goldschmidt-Clermont PJ. Loss of bone marrow-derived vascular progenitor cells leads to inflammation and atherosclerosis. Am Heart J 2003;146:S5–S12.
[31] Goldschmidt-Clermont PJ, Peterson ED. On the memory of a chronic illness. Sci Aging Knowl Environ 2003;2003(45):re8.
[32] Rauscher FM, Goldschmidt-Clermont PJ, Davis BH, Wang T, Gregg D, Ramaswani P, et al. Aging, progenitor cell exhaustion, and atherosclerosis. Circulation 2003;108:457–63.
[33] Gnecchi M, Zhang Z, Ni A, Dzau VJ. Paracrine mechanisms in adult stem cell signaling and therapy. Circ Res 2008;103(11):1204–19.
[34] Suuronen EJ, Price J, Veinot JP, Ascah K, Kapila V, Guo X-W, et al. Comparative effects of mesenchymal progenitor cells, endothelial progenitor cells, or their combination on myocardial infarct regeneration and cardiac function. J Thorac Cardiovasc Surg 2007; 134(5):1249–58.
[35] Uemura R, Xu M, Ahmad N, Ashraf M. Bone marrow stem cells prevent left ventricular remodeling of ischemic heart through paracrine signaling. Circ Res 2006; 98(11):1414–21.
[36] Friedenstein AJ, Chailakhjan RK, Lalykina KS. The development of fibroblast colonies in monolayer cultures of guinea-pig bone marrow and spleen cells. Cell Tissue Kinet 1970;3:393–403.
[37] Lennon D, Caplan A. Isolation of human marrow-derived mesenchymal stem cells. Exp Hematol 2006;34:1604–5.
[38] Beyer Nardi N, da Silva Meirelles L. Mesenchymal stem cells: isolation, in vitro expansion and characterization. Handbook Exp Pharmacol 2006;174:249–82.
[39] Prockop D. Marrow stromal cells as stem cells for nonhematopoietic tissues. Science 1997;276:71–4.
[40] Sethe S, Scutt A, Stolzing A. Aging of mesenchymal stem cells. Ageing Res Rev 2006; 5:91–116.
[41] Pittenger M, Mackay A, Beck S, Jaiswal R, Douglas R, Mosca J, et al. Multilineage potential of adult human mesenchymal stem cell. Science 1999;284:143–7.
[42] Uccelli A, Moretta L, Pistoia V. Mesenchymal stem cells in health and disease. Nat Rev Immunol 2008;8:726–36.
[43] Dominici M, Le Blanc K, Mueller I, Slaper-Cortenbach I, Marini F, Krause D, et al. Minimal criteria for defining multipotent mesenchymal stromal cells. The International Society for Cellular Therapy position statement. Cytotherapy 2006;8(4):315–7.
[44] D'Ippolito G, Diabira S, Howard G, Menei P, Roos B, Schiller P. Marrow-isolated adult multilieage inducible (MIAMI0 cells, a unique population of postnatal young and old human cells with extensive expansion and differentiation potential. J Cell Sci 2004;117:2971–81.
[45] Reyes M, Lund T, Lenvik T, Agular D, Koodie L, Verfaillie C. Purification and ex vivo expansion of postnatal human marrow mesodermal progenitor cells. Blood 2001; 98:2615–25.
[46] Asahara T, Murohara T, Sullivan A, Silver M, van der Zee R, Li T, et al. Isolation of putative progenitor endothelial cells for angiogenesis. Science 1997;275:964–7.

[47] Zhang H, Zhang N, Li M, Fang H, HJin W, Zhao H, et al. Therapeutic angiogenesis of bone marrow mononuclear cells (MNCs) and peripheral blood MNCs: transplantation for ischmic hindlimb. Ann Vasc Surg 2008;22:238–47.

[48] Kinnaird T, Stabile E, Burnett MS, Lee CW, Barr S, Fuchs S, et al. Marrow-derived stromal cells express genes encoding a broad spectrum of arteriogenic cytokines and promote in vitro and in vivo arteriogenesis through paracrine mechanisms. Circ Res 2004;94(5):678–85.

[49] Prather W, Toren A, Meiron M, Ofir R, Tschope C, Horwitz E. The role of placental- derived adherent stromal cell (PLX-PAD) in the treatment of critical limb ischemia. Cytotherapy 2009;11(4):427–34.

[50] Christ O, Lucke K, Imren S, Leung K, Hamilton M, Eaves A, et al. Improved purification of hematopoietic stem cells based on their elevated aldehyde dehydrogenase activity. Haematologica 2007;92(9):1165–72.

[51] Fallon P, Gentry T, Balber AE, Boulware D, Janssen WE, Smilee R, et al. Mobilized peripheral blood SSC^{lo} $ALDH^{br}$ cells have the phenotypic and functional properties of primitive haematopoietic cells and their number correlates with engraftment following autologous transplantation. Br J Haematol 2003;122:99–108.

[52] Gentry T, Foster S, Winstead L, Deibert E, Fiordalisi M, Balber A. Simultaneous isolation of human BM hematopoietic, endothelial and mesenchymal progenitor cells by flow sorting based on aldehyde dehydrogenase activity: implications for cell therapy. Cytotherapy 2007;9(3):259–74.

[53] Perin EC, Silva GV, Chronos N, Mitchell RG, Mendelsohn FO, Gahremanpour A, et al. Abstract 4934 CLI-Bright: a phase i randomized blinded clinical trial comparing the effect of intramuscular injection of autologous bone marrow derived aldehyde dehydrogenase bright cells and mononuclear stem cells in patients with critical limb ischemia. Circulation 2009; 120(18):S1024.

[54] Zhu S, Dong C, Gentry T, Balber AE, Goldschmidt-Clermont PJ. Aldehyde dehydrogenase-positive stem cells from the human bone marrow differentiate into endothelial cells more efficiently than CD133 + /CD34+ endothelial progenitor cells. J Am Coll Card 2005;45(3):398A.

[55] Capoccia BJ, Robson DL, Levac KD, Maxwell DJ, Hohm SA, Neelamkavil MJ, et al. Revascularization of ischemic limbs after transplantation of human bone marrow cells with high aldehyde dehydrogenase activity. Blood 2009;113(21):5340–51.

[56] Kawamoto A, Iwasaki H, Kusano K, Murayama T, Oyamada A, Silver M, et al. CD34-positive cells exhibit increased potency and safety for therapeutic neovascularization after myocardial infarction compared with total mononuclear cells. Circulation 2006;114(20):2163–9.

[57] Canizo M, Lozano F, Gonzalez-Porras J, Barros M, Lopez-Hogado N, Briz E, et al. Peripheral endothelial progenitor cells (CD133+) for therapeutic vasculogenesis in a paitent with critical limb ischemia. One year follow-up. Cytotherapy 2007;9:99–102.

[58] Kudo F, Nishibe T, Nishibe M, Yasuda K. Autologous transplantation of peripheral blood endothelial progenitor cells (CD34+) for therapeutic angiogenesis in patients with critical limb ischemia. Int Angiol 2003;22:344–8.

[59] Tateishi-Yuyama E, Matsubara H, Murohara T, Ikeda U, Shintani S, Masaki H, et al. Therapeutic angiogenesis for patients with limb ischaemia by autologous transplantation of bone-marrow cells: a pilot study and a randomised controlled trial. Lancet 2002; 360(9331):427–35.

[60] Huang P, Yang X, Li S, Wen J, Zhang Y, Ham Z. Randomized comparison of G-CSF-mobilized peripheral blood mononuclear cells versus bone marrow-mononuclear cells

for the treatment of patients with lower limb arteriosclerosis obliterans. Thromb Haemost 2007;98:1335–42.
[61] Mukai N, Akahori T, Komaki M, Li Q, Kanayasu-Toyoda T, Ishii-Watabe A, et al. A comparison of the tube forming potentials of early and late endothelial progenitor cells. Exp Cell Res 2008;314(3):430–40.
[62] Rookmaaker MB, Verhaar MC, Loomans CJM, Verloop R, Peters E, Westerweel PE, et al. CD34+ cells home, proliferate, and participate in capillary formation, and in combination with CD34- cells enhance tube formation in a 3-dimensional matrix. Arterioscler Thromb Vasc Biol 2005;25(9):1843–50.
[63] Zhang S, Zhang P, Guo J, Jia Z, Ma K, Liu Y, et al. Enhanced cytoprotection and angiogenesis by bonemarrow cell transplantation may contribute to improved ischemic myocardial functdion. Eur J Cardiothorac Surg 2004;25:188–95.
[64] Delewi R, Andriessen A, Tijssen JGP, Zijlstra F, Piek JJ, Hirsch A. Impact of intracoronary cell therapy on left ventricular function in the setting of acute myocardial infarction: a meta-analysis of randomised controlled clinical trials. Heart 2013;99(4):225–32.
[65] Jeevanantham V, Butler M, Saad A, Abdel-Latif A, Zuba-Surma EK, Dawn B. Adult bone marrow cell therapy improves survival and induces long-term improvement in cardiac parameters: a systematic review and meta-analysis. Circulation 2012;126(5):551–68.
[66] Jeevanantham V, Butler M, Saad A, Dawn B, Abdel-Latif A, Zuba-Surma EK. Response to letter regarding article, "Adult bone marrow cell therapy improves survival and induces long-term improvement in cardiac parameters: a systematic review and meta-analysis". Circulation 2013;127(15):e548.
[67] Zimmet H, Porapakkham P, Porapakkham P, Sata Y, Haas SJ, Itescu S, et al. Short- and long-term outcomes of intracoronary and endogenously mobilized bone marrow stem cells in the treatment of ST-segment elevation myocardial infarction: a meta-analysis of randomized control trials. Eur J Heart Fail 2012;14(1):91–105.
[68] Li TS, Cheng K, Malliaras K, Smith RR, Zhang Y, Sun B, et al. Direct comparison of different stem cell types and subpopulations reveals superior paracrine potency and myocardial repair efficacy with cardiosphere-derived cells. J Am Coll Cardiol 2012;59(10):942–53.
[69] Dubois C, Liu X, Claus P, Marsboom G, Pokreisz P, Vandenwijngaert S, et al. Differential effects of progenitor cell populations on left ventricular remodeling and myocardial neovascularization after myocardial infarction. J Am Coll Cardiol 2010;55(20):2232–43.
[70] Armiñán A, Gandía C, García-Verdugo JM, Lledó E, Trigueros C, Ruiz-Saurí A, et al. Mesenchymal stem cells provide better results than hematopoietic precursors for the treatment of myocardial infarction. J Am Coll Cardiol 2010;55(20):2244–53.
[71] Iwase T, Nagaya N, Fujii T, Itoh T, Murakami S, Matsumoto T, et al. Comparison of angiogenic potency between mesenchymal stem cells and mononuclear cells in a rat model of hindlimb ischemia. 2005;66(3):543–551.
[72] Shichinohe H, Kuroda S, Maruichi K, Osanai T, Sugiyama T, Chiba Y, et al. Bone marrow stromal cells and bone marrow-derived mononuclear cells: which are suitable as cell source of transplantation for mice infarct brain? Neuropathology 2010;30(2):113–22.
[73] Trachtenberg B, Velazquez DL, Williams AR, McNiece I, Fishman J, Nguyen K, et al. Rationale and design of the transendocardial injection of autologous human cells (bone marrow or mesenchymal) in chronic ischemic left ventricular dysfunction and heart failure secondary to myocardial infarction (TAC-HFT) trial: a randomized, double-blind, placebo-controlled study of safety and efficacy. Am Heart J 2011;161(3):487–93.
[74] Heldman AW, DiFede DL, Fishman JE, et al. Transendocardial mesenchymal stem cells and mononuclear bone marrow cells for ischemic cardiomyopathy: the tac-hft randomized trial. JAMA 2014;311(1):62–73.

[75] Lu D, Chen B, Liang Z, Deng W, Jiang Y, Li S, et al. Comparison of bone marrow mesenchymal stem cells with bone marrow-derived mononuclear cells for treatment of diabetic critical limb ischemia and foot ulcer: a double-blind, randomized, controlled trial. Diabetes Res Clin Pract 2011;92(1):26–36.

[76] Powell RJ. Update on clinical trials evaluating the effect of biologic therapy in patients with critical limb ischemia. J Vasc Surg 2012;56(1):264–6.

[77] Raval Z, Losordo DW. Cell therapy of peripheral arterial disease: from experimental findings to clinical trials. Circ Res 2013;112(9):1288–302.

[78] Heeschen C, Lehmann R, Honold J, Assmus B, Aicher A, Walter DH, et al. Profoundly reduced neovascularization capacity of bone marrow mononuclear cells derived from patients with chronic ischemic heart disease. Circulation 2004;109:1615–22.

[79] Nikol S, Baumgartner I, Van Belle E, Diehm C, Visona A, Capogrossi MC, et al. Therapeutic angiogenesis with intramuscular NV1FGF improves amputation-free survival in patients with critical limb ischemia. Mol Ther 2008;16(5):972–8.

[80] Belch JF, Hiatt WR, Baumgartner I, Driver VR, Nikol S, Norgren L, et al. Effect of fibroglast growth factor NV1FGF on amputation and death: a randomized placebo-controlled trial of gene therapy in critical limb ischaemia. Lancet 2011;377:1929–37.

[81] Duong Van Huyen J, Smadja D, Bruneval P, Gaussem P, Dal-Cortivo L, Julia P, et al. Bone marrow-derived mononuclear cell implantation improves endothelium-dpendent vasodilation in patients with limb ischemia. Circulation 2008;109:1215–8.

[82] Baumgartner I, Chronos N, Comerota A, Henry T, Pasquet J-P, Finiels F, et al. Local gene transfer and expression following intramuscular administration of FGF-1 plasmid DNA in patients with critical limb ischemia. Mol Ther 2009;17(5):914–21.

[83] Walter DH, Krankenberg H, Balzer JO, Kalka C, Baumgartner I, Schlüter M, et al. Intraarterial administration of bone marrow mononuclear cells in patients with critical limb ischemia: a randomized-start, Placebo-Controlled Pilot Trial (PROVASA). Circulation 2011; 4(1):26–37.

[84] Bartsch T, Brehm M, Zeus T, Kögler G, Wernet P, Strauer B. Transplantation of autologous mononuclear bone marrow stem cells in patients with peripheral arterial disease (The TAM-PAD study). Clin Res Cardiol 2007;96(12):891–9. English.

[85] Losordo DW, Kibbe MR, Mendelsohn F, Marston W, Driver VR, Sharafuddin M, et al. A randomized, controlled pilot study of autologous CD34+ cell therapy for critical limb ischemia. Circulation 2012;5(6):821–30.

[86] Cobellis G, Silvestroni A, Lillo S, Sica G, Botti C, Maione C, et al. Long-term effects of repeated autologous transplantation of bone marrow cells in patients affected by peripheral arterial disease. Bone Marrow Transplant 2008;42(10):667–72.

[87] Franz RW, Parks A, Shah KJ, Hankins T, Hartman JF, Wright ML. Use of autologous bone marrow mononuclear cell implantation therapy as a limb salvage procedure in patients with severe peripheral arterial disease. J Vasc Surg 2009;50(6):1378–2130.

[88] Franz RW, Shah KJ, Johnson JD, Pin RH, Parks AM, Hankins T, et al. Short- to mid-term results using autologous bone-marrow mononuclear cell implantation therapy as a limb salvage procedure in patients with severe peripheral arterial disease. Vasc Endovasc Surg 2011;45(5):398–406.

[89] Higashi Y, Kimura M, Hara K, Noma K, Jitsuiki D, Nakagawa K, et al. Autologous bone-marrow mononuclear cell implantation improves endothelium-dependent vasodilation in patients with limb ischemia. Circulation 2004;109(10):1215–8.

[90] Ishida A, Ohya Y, Sakuda H, Ohshiro K, Higashiuesato Y, Nakaema M, et al. Autologous peripheral blood mononuclear cell implantation for patients with peripheral arterial disease improves limb ischemia. Circulation J 2005;69(10):1260–5.

[91] Kamata Y, Takahashi Y, Iwamoto M, Matsui K, Murakami Y, Muroi K, et al. Local implantation of autologous mononuclear cells from bone marrow and peripheral blood for treatment of ischaemic digits in patients with connective tissue diseases. Rheumatology 2007;46(5):882–4.

[92] Lara-Hernandez R, Lozano-Vilardell P, Blanes P, Torreguitart-Mirada N, Galmés A, Besalduch J. Safety and efficacy of therapeutic angiogenesis as a novel treatment in patients with critical limb ischemia. Ann Vasc Surg 2010;24(2):287–94.

[93] Lenk K, Adams V, Lurz P, Erbs S, Linke A, Gielen S, et al. Therapeutical potential of blood-derived progenitor cells in patients with peripheral arterial occlusive disease and critical limb ischaemia. 2005; 26(18):1903–1909.

[94] Motukuru V, Surech KR, Vivekanand V, raj S, Girja KR. Therapeutic angiogenesis in Buerger's disease (thromboangiitis obliterans) patients with critical limb ischemia by autologous transplantation of bone marrow mononuclear cells. J Vasc Surg 2008;48:53S–60S.

[95] Ruiz-Salmeron R, de la Cuesta-Diaz A, Constantino-Bermejo M, Perez-Camacho I, Marcos-Sanchez F, Hmadcha A, et al. Angiographic demonstration of neoangiogenesis after intra-arterial infusion of autologous bone marrow mononuclear cells in diabetic patients with critical limb ischemia. Cell Transplant 2011;20:1629–39.

[96] Saito Y, Sasaki K-i, Katsuda Y, Murohara T, Takeshita Y, Okazaki T, et al. Effect of autologous bone-marrow cell transplantation on ischemic ulcer in patients with Buerger's disease. Circulation J 2007;71(8):1187–92.

[97] Van Huyen J-PD, Smadja DM, Bruneval P, Gaussem P, Dal-Cortivo L, Julia P, et al. Bone marrow-derived mononuclear cell therapy induces distal angiogenesis after local injection in critical leg ischemia. Mod Pathol 2008;21(7):837–46.

[98] Van Tongeren R, Hamming J, Fibbe W, Van Weel V, Grerichs S, Stiggelbout A, et al. Intramuscular or combined intramuscular/intra-arterial administration of bone marrow mononuclear cells a clinical trial in patients with advanced limb ischemia. J Cardiovasc Surg 2008;49:51–8.

[99] Matoba S, Tatsumi T, Murohara T, Imaizumi T, Katsuda Y, Ito M, et al. Long-term clinical outcome after intramuscular implantation of bone marrow mononuclear cells (Therapeutic Angiogenesis by Cell Transplantation [TACT] trial) in patients with chronic limb ischemia. Am Heart J 2008;156(5):1010–8.

[100] Duong Van Huyen J, Smadja D, Bruneval P, Guaussem P, Dal-Cortivo L, Julia P, et al. Bone marrow-derived mononuclear cell therapy induces distal angiogenesis after local injeciton in critical leg ischemia. Mod Pathol 2008;21:837–46.

[101] Losordo DW, Henry TD, Davidson C, Lee JS, Costa MA, Bass T, et al. Intramyocardial, autologous CD34+ cell therapy for refractory angina. Circ Res 2011;109(4):428–36.

[102] Huang P, Li S, Han M, Xiao Z, Yang R, Han ZC. Autologous transplantation of granulocyte colony-stimulating factor-mobilized peripheral blood mononuclear cells improves critical limb ischemia in diabetes. Diabetes Care 2005;28(9):2155–60.

[103] Huang PP, Yang XF, Li SZ, Wen JC, Zhang Y, Han ZC. Autologous transplantation of peripheral blood stem cells as an effective therapeutic approach for severe arteriosclerosis obliterans of lower extremeties. Thromb Haemost 2004;91:606–9.

[104] Huang PP, Yang XF, Li SZ, Wen JC, Zhang Y, Han ZC. Randomised comparison of G-CSF-mobilized peripheral blood mononuclear cells versus bone marrow-mononuclear cells for the treatment of patients with lower limb arteriosclerosis obliterans. Thromb Haemost 2007;98(12):1335–42. En.

[105] Fadini GP, Agostini C, Avogaro A. Autologous stem cell therapy for peripheral arterial disease: meta-analysis and systematic review of the literature. Atherosclerosis 2010; 209(1):10–7.

[106] Napoli C, Farzati B, Sica V, et al. Beneficial effects of autologous bone marrow cell infusion and antioxidants/L-arginine in patients with chronic critical limb ischemia. Eur J Cardiovasc Prev Rehabil 2008;15:709–18.

[107] Bartel RL, Carmer C, Ledford K, Longcore A, Parrish C, Stem T, et al. The Aastrom experience. Stem Cell Res Ther 2012;3:26.

[108] Marston W, Powell RJ, Dall'Olmo C, Guzman R, Moore C, Martinez J, et al. Patient-specific cellular therapy (Ixmyelocel-T) is safe and improves time to treatment failure in patients with critical limb ischemia and no revascularization options. Circulation 2011;124:A8547.

[109] Perin EC, Silva G, Gahremanpour A, Canales J, Zheng Y, Cabreira-Hansen MG, et al. A randomized, controlled study of autologous therapy with bone marrow–derived aldehyde dehydrogenase bright cells in patients with critical limb ischemia. Catheter Cardiovasc Interv 2011;78(7):1060–7.

[110] Perin EC, Murphy M, Cooke JP, Moyé L, Henry TD, Bettencourt J, et al. Rationale and design for PACE: patients with intermittent claudication injected with ALDH bright cells. Am Heart J 2015;168(5). 667-73.e2.

[111] https://http://www.clinicaltrials.gov/ct2/show/NCT01558908?term=medistem&rank=2.

[112] Asahara T, Masuda H, Takahashi T, Kalka C, Pastore C, Silver M, et al. Bone marrow origin of endothelial progenitor cells responsible for postnatal vasculogenesis in physiological and pathological neovascularization. Circulation 1999;85:221–8.

[113] Takahashi T, Kalka C, Masuda H, Chen D, Silver M, Kearney M, et al. Ischemia-, and cytokine-induced mobilization of bone marrow-derived endothelial cell progenitor cells for neovascularization. Nat Med 1999;5:434–8.

[114] Kokkinos P, Myers J, Faselis C, Panagiotakos DB, Doumas M, Pittaras A, et al. Exercise capacity and mortality in older men: a 20-year follow-up study. Circulation 2010; 122(8):790–7.

[115] Myers J, Prakash M, Froelicher V, Do D, Partington S, Atwood JE. Exercise capacity and mortality among men referred for exercise testing. New Engl J Med 2002; 346(11):793–801.

[116] Povsic TJ, Junge C, Nada A, Schatz RA, Harrington RA, Davidson CJ, et al. A phase 3, randomized, double-blinded, active-controlled, unblinded standard of care study assessing the efficacy and safety of intramyocardial autologous CD34+ cell administration in patients with refractory angina: design of the RENEW study. Am Heart J 2013;165(6). 854-61.e2.

[117] Felker GM, Maisel AS. A global rank end point for clinical trials in acute heart failure. Circulation 2010;3(5):643–6.

[118] Jaski BE, Jessup ML, Mancini DM, Cappola TP, Pauly DF, Greenberg B, et al. Calcium upregulation by percutaneous administration of gene therapy in cardiac disease (CUPID Trial), a first-in-human phase 1/2 clinical trial. J Card Fail 2009;15(3):171–81.

[119] Teerlink JR, Metra M, Felker GM, Ponikowski P, Voors AA, Weatherley BD, et al. Relaxin for the treatment of patients with acute heart failure (Pre-RELAX-AHF): a multicentre, randomised, placebo-controlled, parallel-group, dose-finding phase IIb study. Lancet 2009;373(9673):1429–39.

[120] Baumgartner I, Thoeny H, Kummer O, Roefke C, Skjelsvik C, Boesch C, et al. Leg ischemia: assessment with MR angiogrpahy and spectroscopy. Radiology 2005;234:833–41.

[121] Greve JM, Chico TJ, Goldman H, Bunting S, Peale FV, Daugherty A, et al. Magnetic resonance angiography reveals therapeutic enlargement of collateral vessels induced by VEGF in a murine model of peripheral arterial disease. J Magn Reson 2006;24(5):1124–32.

[122] Leong-Poi H. Molecular imaging using contrast-enhanced ultrasound: evaluation of angiogenesis and cell therapy. Cardiovasc Res 2009;94:190–200.

[123] Oses P, Renault M-A, Chauvel R, Leroux L, Allières C, Séguy B, et al. Mapping 3-dimensional neovessel organization steps using micro-computed tomography in a murine model of hindlimb ischemia–brief report. Arterioscler Thromb Vasc Biol 2009;29(12):2090–2.
[124] Miyamoto M, Yasutake M, Takano H, Takagi H, Takagi G, Mizuno H, et al. Therapeutic angiogenesis by autologous bone marrow cell implantation for refractory chronic peripheral arterial disease using assessment of neovascularization by 99mTc-tetrafosmin (TF) perfusion scintigraphy. Cell Transplant 2004;13:429–37.

Chapter 5

Endothelial Progenitor Cells for Vascular Medicine

H. Masuda, MD, PhD*, A. Kawamoto, MD, PhD**, M. Ii, MD, PhD†, T. Asahara, MD, PhD*

**Department of Regenerative Medicine Science, Tokai University School of Medicine, Isehara, Kanagawa, Japan; **Unit of Regenerative Medicine, Institute of Biomedical Research and Innovation, Chuo-ku, Kobe, Japan; †Department of Pharmacology, Group of Translational Stem Cell Research, Osaka Medical College, Takatsuki, Osaka, Japan*

ENDOTHELIAL PROGENITOR CELL

Endothelial progenitor cells (EPCs) have been isolated for the first time from adult peripheral blood (PB) in 1997 [1], and could be further shown to derive from bone marrow (BM) and other tissues, representing a highly proangiogenic pool of cells prone to accumulate into foci of physiological and pathological neovascularization [2,3] exhibiting characteristics, usually associated with common stem/progenitor cells. BM-derived EPCs can be home to sites of neovascularization and may even differentiate into endothelial cells (ECs) in situ, a mechanism consistent with "vasculogenesis", a critical paradigm well described for embryonic vascularization, but only recently proposed for the adult organism, with a possible reservoir of stem/progenitor cells contributing to postnatal vascular formation, vascular regeneration, and tissue homeostasis (Fig. 5.1). The discovery of EPCs has therefore radically changed our understanding of adult blood vessel formation, specifically in ischemic tissues. The following review will highlight the potential value of EPCs for therapeutic vasculogenesis in ischemic diseases, focusing particularly on one of the most pressing and still unresolved issues in the field, the proper definition of EPC.

Definition of EPCs

Endothelial progenitor cells or "EPCs" were originally described as blood bound cells with the ability to differentiate into the endothelial lineage [4]. Believed to be a "progenitor cell," EPCs were thought to be able to reside in their immature state and upon the encounter of appropriate stimuli to migrate, proliferate, or differentiate into a more mature lineage, capable of either direct contribution

Regenerative Medicine for Peripheral Artery Disease. http://dx.doi.org/10.1016/B978-0-12-801344-1.00005-X

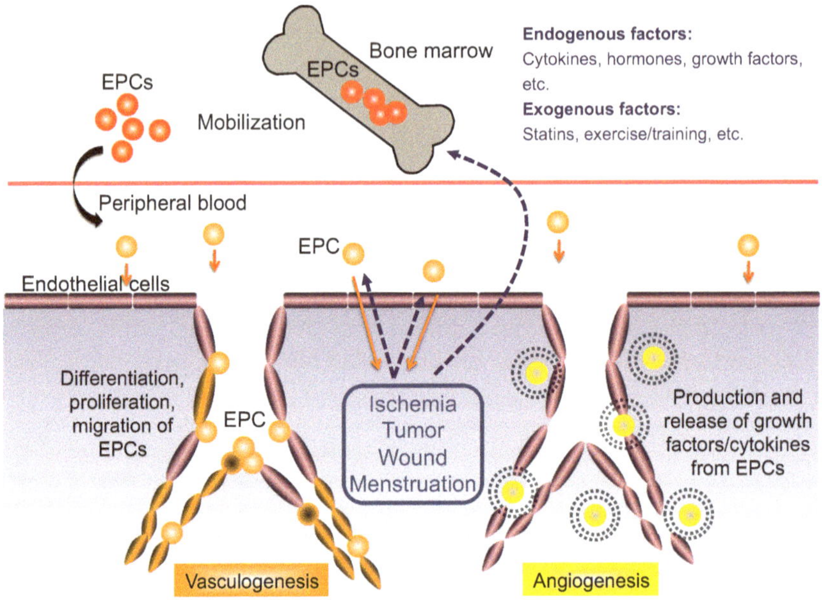

FIGURE 5.1 **Role of EPCs in angio-/vasculogenesis.** The concept of "angiogenesis" is characterized by the proliferation and migration of preexisting endothelial cells (ECs) forming new vessels in response to endogenous or exogenous stimuli (right in the figure). In contrast, a variety of factors released from the jeopardized tissue or surrounding areas affect the BM remotely and mobilize EPCs from the BM into circulation. EPCs recruit (home) to the site of injury and participate in neovascularization, by differentiating, proliferating, and migrating into the newly forming vasculature, confirming the concept of "vasculogenesis" (left in the figure).

to or at least support of regenerative processes, namely the regeneration of the injured cardiovascular system.

EPCs are currently believed to be represented by the following hallmarks: (1) the ability for endothelial lineage commitment, and the acquisition of an EC specific or "EC-equivalent" phenotype, (2) initial immatureness, while preserving the competence to differentiate, indicated by a primitive progenitor cell phenotype and the (partial) lack of mature EC markers, and (3) the presence of proangiogenic and vasculogenic properties, with a strong biological activity toward neovascular formation resulting in functional recovery and regeneration of the injured vascular system. Besides these general hallmarks, EPCs can be distinguished and subdivided into various categories.

Tissue EPCs Versus Circulating EPCs

On the basis of their in vivo classification, one can distinguish between "tissue EPCs" and "circulating EPCs." Tissue EPCs are characterized by their adhesive nature and the fact that they can be isolated directly from organ tissues, representing either EPCs in the wake of differentiation originating from the

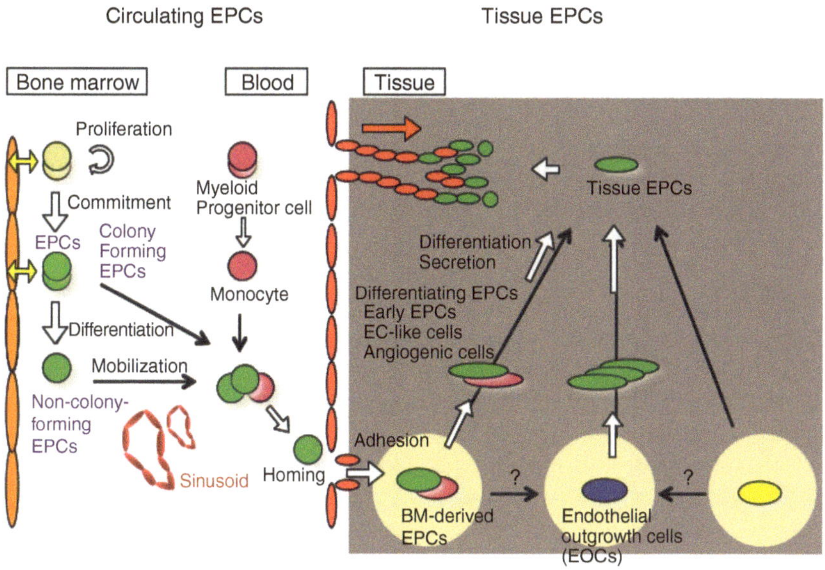

FIGURE 5.2 Kinetics of circulating EPCs and tissue EPCs. The relationship among EPCs in the BM, blood, and organ tissues, and their differentiation cascade is represented in the figure. HPP, high proliferative; LPP, low proliferative; and ECFC, endothelial colony-forming cell.

circulation, so called “homed-down” circulatory EPCs, endothelial outgrowth cells (EOCs) of a yet to be defined origin, or cells of the endothelial lineage which are directly derived from organ-based stem and progenitor cells such as cardiac stem cells [5], neural stem cells [6], myogenic stem cells, or mesenchymal stem cells [7] (Fig. 5.2). On the other hand, circulating EPCs are cellular components of blood which can be isolated from peripheral blood (PB), umbilical cord blood (UCB), BM, and from organs or organ blood vessels. Circulating EPCs emerge as floating, nonadhesive cells present in and moving throughout the circulatory system. A “suspended, nonattaching blood cell state” is therefore most characteristic for circulating EPCs which can mobilize and be recruited from preservative and educational niches in the BM into the blood stream, and home to sites of ischemic and/or vascular distress, contributing to the regeneration of the target tissue by transforming into adhesive EPCs.

Hematopoietic EPCs Versus Nonhematopoietic EPCs

Hematopoietic EPCs (h-EPCs)

Circulating EPCs can be subdivided into two main categories, hematopoietic lineage EPCs (h-EPCs) and nonhematopoietic lineage EPCs (nh-EPCs) (Fig. 5.2). The h-EPCs originate from BM and represent a provasculogenic subpopulation of hematopoietic stem cells (HSCs). The h-EPCs can enter circulation upon stimulation as cellular components of blood, compromising a possibly heterogeneous cell population, represented by, for example, colony-forming EPCs, non-colony-forming "differentiating" EPCs, myeloid EPCs or angiogenic cells etc. The nh-EPCs are not HSC-derived cells, which can be isolated from blood or tissue samples via the help of adhesive cell-culture techniques and distinguished by their rather obvious EC(-like) phenotype. The origin of nh-EPCs remains to be clarified, but they are generally thought to be derived from nonhematopoietic tissue prone lineage stem cells or organ blood vessels.

The h-EPCs can be further subdivided into three distinct classes. The first class is represented by EPCs which can be classified as direct descendant of HSCs, which can form immature hematopoietic-like EPC colonies and commit into circulating EC-like cells. The second class is represented by myeloid cells derived from myeloid progenitors, already committed to the myeloid lineage, but still capable to differentiate into EC-like cells, mimicking an endothelial cell phenotype. The third type is represented by cells, loosely termed circulating angiogenic cells (CACs), which can give rise to EC-like cells and contribute to neovascularization mainly by the secretion of proangiogenic growth factors. The characterization and identification of HSC-derived EPCs are tightly linked to and associated with the methods and markers already applied in the hematopoietic field. EPCs and HSCs can both be isolated using antibodies against various cell surface markers, including membrane receptors such as CD34, CD133, Flk-1/KDR, CXCR4, CD105 (Endoglin) for human samples [1,8–13] and receptors such as c-Kit [14], Sca-1 [15,16], and CD34 [14,17] in combination with Flk-1 (VEGFR2) in case of mouse samples. Nevertheless, the identification of a unique combination of receptors specific and selective for primary EPCs, enabling an unambiguous distinction between EPCs and HSCs is still missing. The introduction of a definitive assay system capable of clearly distinguishing between EPCs and HSCs, thus enabling the identification of the long-sought precise primary EPC phenotype, is highly anticipated but still missing.

Colony-Forming EPCs Versus Non-Colony-Forming EPCs

Colony-Forming EPCs

A novel recently developed EPC colony-forming assay (EPC-CFA) system, capable to address and overcome most of the aforementioned limitations of the classical assay systems, is challenging several of the predominant classical opinions about EPCs, and enabling a differential hierarchic view on EPCs that was missing until now. We recently reported one of the first examples of such an assay system, initially designed to work with mouse samples. c-Kit^{+}/Sca-1^{+}/Lineage negative (KSL) cells were used as a putative murine hematopoietic EPC-enriched cell population, allowing the identification of two clearly distinguishable types of colonies (small and large colonies) that in turn correspond to two distinct EPC populations, primitive (small) and definitive (large) EPCs, respectively [18–20] (Fig. 5.3). The concept of an EPC-CFA was recently

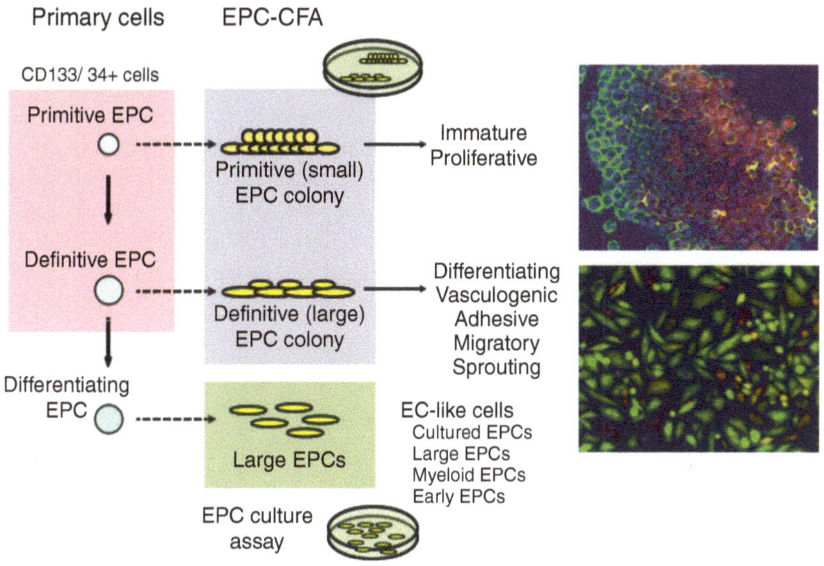

FIGURE 5.3 Differentiation cascade of blood EPCs and in vitro EPC assay system. (1) Heterogeneous cell populations including myeloid cell-, lymphoid cell-, and EPC-aggregates are assessed by Hill's colony assay system; (2) relatively purified EPC-rich cell populations including primitive (small) EPCs and definitive (large) EPCs are assessed by EPC-CFA; and (3) small/large EPCs, monocytic EPCs, and angiogenic monocyte/macrophages are assessed by culture EPC assay system.

introduced and further developed for analysis of human EPC samples (Masuda et al, unpublished data). The EPC-CFA enables hereby not only the EPC-colony formation analysis of single and/or bulk cells from EPC-enriched arbitrary fractions or nonselected cell populations but also allows the cell fate analysis of primary and/or suspension culture cultivated single and/or bulk cells. It can further be easily combined with a classical HPC colony assay system, thus allowing a direct and comprehensive elucidation of the differences and similarities between EPCs and HPCs via the clarification of the cell fate of each cell type. The use of such an EPC-CFA allows not only the elucidation of a possible but so far elusive differentiation hierarchy of EPCs but also identification and characterization of the parameters associated with proliferation, commitment, and differentiation of EPCs in vitro and in vivo.

Indeed, application of EPC-CFA on human CD34+ or CD133+ stem/progenitor cells enabled the identification of small and large distinct colony types each derived from a single cell, small-EPCs and large-EPCs, respectively (Fig. 5.3). Small-EPCs showed a higher rate of proliferative activity with a higher number of cells being in the S-phase, when compared to large-EPCs. Interestingly, large-EPCs showed a significantly higher rate of vasculogenic activity with overall increased potential for cell adhesion and tube-like structure formation in vitro as well as a high in vivo de novo blood-vessel-forming activity following transplantation of these cells into a murine ischemic hindlimb model, as compared to small-EPCs. In contrast to small-EPCs, large-EPCs did not form secondary colonies but gave rise to isolated endothelial cell (EC)-like cells when reseeded. Due to the observed in vitro (by FACS analysis) and in vivo characteristics of these colony types, small-EPCs were further characterized and believed to represent "primitive EPCs," a highly immature and proliferative population of cells, compared to large-EPCs which are believed to represent "definitive EPCs," cells prone to differentiate and promote vasculogenesis.

Non-Colony-Forming EPCs

The widely used "classical EPC culture assay" systems are characterized by the appearance of adhesive endothelial lineage (-like) cells upon conditioning of PB- or BM-derived mononuclear cells with endothelial growth factor–supplemented media [21–23]. These overall reproducible and standardized assay systems were used for the characterization of a wide range of EPCs, ranging from "cultured EPCs" [21,23–26], "EC-like cells" [27], "early EPCs" [26,28,29] to so-called "circulating angiogenic cells" [30,31], which generally do not form colonies under conventional endothelial differentiation conditions.

Cultured EPCs are often called "EC-like cells" due to the expression of certain endothelial features such as: (1) the expression of certain endothelial lineage marker genes/proteins such as CD31, Flk-1/KDR, Flt-1, VE-cadherin, Tie-2, vWF, (2) an EC-like bioactivity, characterized by their capacity to migrate toward an angiogenic growth factor gradient or to support the formation of or incorporate into tube-like structures, and (3) their direct/indirect contribution to the formation of new blood vessels in ischemic tissues after in vivo transplantation. Other characteristics of these cells also cover nonendothelial features such as (1) hematopoietic cell marker expression, for example, CD45 or CD14 up to 2 weeks in culture, (2) loss of EC monolayer formation, and (3) reduction of their proliferative activity in culture similar to cultured human endothelial cells, for example, HUVEC [21,24,26]. The obvious discrepancies between differentiating EPCs and differentiated ECs characterized by a lack of certain endothelial specific markers and properties of EC-like cells and the obvious diminished EPC differentiation capacity into totally differentiated EC phenotype in vitro have been discussed for years and still remain to be clarified.

Role of EPCs in Postnatal Neovascularization

Direct EPC Contribution to Neovascularization

Neovascularization in the adult organism was longtime believed to be solely based on the mechanism of "angiogenesis," a term used to circumscribe the process of new vessel formation, via in situ proliferation and migration of preexisting ECs [32]. The identification of EPCs lead to a paradigm shift, introducing "vasculogenesis" previously only with embryonic development associated process as a novel mechanism for vessel formation and vascular regeneration into the adult setting. In the context of EPC biology, "vasculogenesis" covers the de novo formation of blood vessel via in situ migration, proliferation, differentiation, and/or incorporation of BM-derived EPCs into regenerating vasculature [2] (Fig. 5.1). The incorporation of BM-derived EPCs into foci of physiological and pathological neovascularization has been demonstrated in various animal models, albeit remaining a still controversial topic in the field of EPC biology with several contradicting reports being published so far. Nevertheless, one well-established model, allowing the detection of BM-derived EPCs, utilizes transplantation of BM cells from transgenic mice in which LacZ is expressed under the regulation of an EC lineage-specific promoter, such as Flk-1 or Tie-2 (Flk-1/LacZ/BMT, Tie-2/LacZ/BMT) into wild-type control mice, followed by their use as a base for several different ischemic injury models. Utilizing such a model, it has been shown that BM-derived Flk-1- and/or Tie-2-expressing endothelial lineage cells can localize to vascular structures during tumor growth [2,33], wound healing [34], skeletal [2] and cardiac ischemia [35,36], corneal neovascularization [37], and endometrial remodeling following hormone-induced ovulation [2,33]. On the other hand, tissue-specific stem/progenitor cells with the potency to differentiate into myocytes or endothelial cells were also isolated from skeletal muscle tissue in murine hindlimb, although the origin of the cells remains to be clarified [38]. This finding suggests that the origin of EPCs may not be limited to BM, for example, tissue specific stem/progenitor cells may possibly provide "in situ EPCs" as already discussed previously. Regardless of the origin of EPCs, they undoubtedly play a significant role contributing to neovascularization via vasculogenesis in ischemic tissues.

Indirect EPC Contribution to Neovascularization

Albeit the well-established model of EPC action during neovascularization, that is the "direct participation/integration into the forming neovasculature of ischemic organs via vasculogenesis," EPCs migrating to distressed tissues and organs urgently requiring vascular regeneration do not always participate in the formation of the neovasculature but rather "stay out" residing in the interstitial tissue. These tissue-bound "resting EPCs" produce a variety of proangiogenic cytokines and growth factors, promoting proliferation and migration of preexisting ECs, activating angiogenesis, and contributing "indirectly" to vascular regeneration and the reestablishment of tissue homeostasis (Figs. 5.1 and 5.2). Thus, EPCs do not only work via the activation and support of "vasculogenesis" but may also be major players involved in the activation and mediation of "angiogenesis", the process of new vessel formation, via in situ proliferation and migration of preexisting ECs [32]. This paracrine aspect of EPC activity reflecting their indirect contribution to neovascularization was confirmed by us and other groups, demonstrating the presence of various cytokines and other secreted proangiogenic factors in EPCs such as VEGF, HGF, Ang-1, SDF-1α, IGF-1, and eNOS/iNOS [35,39]. Growth factors such as VEGF and HGF can promote EC proliferation inducing/propagating angiogenesis, whereas, for example, Ang-1 can stabilize and help the maturation of immature new vessels forming in ischemic tissue when EPCs are transplanted. Nitric oxide (NO) synthases, eNOS, and iNOS, contribute as vasodilators to the maintenance of microcirculatory activity and blood flow in ischemic tissues, thus also influencing overall tissue/organ regeneration and recovery. SDF-1α, a potent chemoattractant is released from recruited EPCs, which leads to further recruitment of additional EPCs triggering a self-sustained and self-supporting mechanism promoting vascular regeneration. IGF-1, a potent antiapoptotic factor, which is another example for a growth factor that can be released by EPCs, is for instance cardioprotective preventing cardiac cell apoptosis affected by an ischemic insult via the activation of the AKT signaling pathway. In summary, EPCs can mediate tissue-protective effects and contribute to neovascularization in ischemic tissues via production of "indirect working supportive" factors (Fig. 5.1).

EPC-BASED THERAPEUTIC ANGIOGENESIS

Since EPCs were first described more than a decade ago, we and other groups focused especially on the regenerative potential of these progenitor cells trying to unravel and understand their unique properties and characteristics with the ultimate goal to translate this knowledge and to improve the clinical applicability/efficacy of these cells in the fight against cardiovascular diseases. The transplantation of blood/BM derived vasculogenic progenitor cells, of EPCs, believed to act like classical progenitor cells, capable of in vitro expansion and differentiation, as well as in vivo migration, proliferation, differentiation, and functional contribution to the newly forming vasculature and overall tissue regeneration opened in this regard unprecedented opportunities for the treatment of ischemic diseases, which thus far was bound to and limited by the classic paradigm of angiogenesis, marking the beginning of a new era in tissue regeneration previously not believed to be possible.

EPC Transplantation in Animal Models

It was shown that therapeutic approaches utilizing culture-expanded EPCs could successfully promote neovascularization and regeneration of ischemic tissues, even when administered as "sole therapy," that is, in the absence of other supportive proangiogenic growth factors. Such a "supply-side" version of therapeutic neovascularization, in which the substrate (EPCs/ECs) rather than ligand (growth factor) comprises the therapeutic tool, was first reported for the intravenous transplantation of human PB-derived cultured EPCs into immunodeficient mice with hindlimb ischemia [24]. These experimental findings proved that exogenously administered EPCs could restore impaired neovascularization in a murine ischemic hindlimb model. A similar study in which human culture-expanded EPCs were transplanted in a nude rat myocardial ischemia model demonstrated that transplanted EPCs recruited to ischemic myocardium and were able to differentiate into ECs in sites of neovascularization. These findings were consistent with the observed preservation of left ventricular (LV) function and a reduction in infraction size [40,41]. Another study in which human cord blood-derived EPCs were transplanted in a nude rat hindlimb ischemia model also demonstrated similar findings with enhanced neovascularization in ischemic tissues [25].

Recently, several groups have explored the therapeutic potential of CD34+ cells as a possible EPC-enriched fraction. As described previously, a clear distinction between HSCs and EPCs with the current available methodology in many cases is not possible; nonetheless is the use of the "hematopoietic" cell-surface marker CD34, for the isolation/enrichment of EPCs is a widely used approach in the field of EPC biology. Shatteman et al. transplanted freshly isolated human CD34+ cells into diabetic nude mice with hindlimb ischemia, and showed significant blood-flow recovery in ischemic limbs [42]. Kocher et al. infused freshly isolated human CD34+ cells into a nude rat model of myocardial ischemia, and observed preservation of LV function and inhibition of cardiac apoptosis [43]. Dose-dependent contribution of CD34+ cells to LV functional recovery and neovascularization in ischemic myocardium has also been demonstrated by Iwasaki et al. [44].

EPC Transplantation in Clinical Trials

Numerous clinical trials are now on going and trying to elucidate the therapeutic effects of EPCs seen in animal models on ischemic diseases, utilizing a broad range of cells which are all believed to consist of or contain, to a certain extent, EPCs and/or pro-vasculogenic/angiogenic cell populations [45,46]. Excellent in-depth reviews summarizing the cells, conditions as well as the therapeutic outcome, efficacy, and safety of the applied strategies are available [47–49] (Table 5.1) (Fig. 5.4).

One example for such a clinical study utilizing EPCs is our reported phase-I/II clinical trial regarding the intramuscular transplantation of autologous and G-CSF-mobilized CD34+ cells in patients with intractable critical limb ischemia (CLI) [50] (Fig. 5.5). The first-in man trial was conducted as a prospective, multicenter, single-blind, and dose-escalation study since 2002 in our institute. G-CSF was used to efficiently mobilize BM-EPCs into the PB, and the mobilized CD34+ cells were isolated as an EPC-enriched fraction. In all subjects, primary endpoint of efficacy score at week 12 was positive, indicating improvement of lower limb ischemia after cell therapy. In addition, both subjective and objective parameters of lower-limb ischemia such as toe brachial pressure index

TABLE 5.1 Clinical Trials for Ischemic Diseases with EPCs

Trial name/author	Disease type	Number of patients (T/C)	EPC type	Study design	Outcome	References
TOPCARE-AMI	AMI	30/29	PB-/BM-derived Cultured EPCs	RT	Effective	[70]
Bartunek et al.	AMI	19/16	CD133	RT	Effective	[71]
Li et al.	AMI	35/35	Gm-PB-CD34	Cohort	Effective	[72]
Tatsumi et al.	AMI	36/18	PB-MNC	Cohort	Effective	[73]
Dobert et al.	AMI	11/15	PB-/BM-derived Cultured EPCs	Cohort	Effective	[74]
Stamm et al.	RMI	46/9	CD133	NRT	Effective	[75,76]
Ahmadi et al.	RMI	18/9	CD133	NRT	Effective	[77]
Balogh et al.	RMI	8/18	CD34	NRT	Inconclu-sive	[78]
Erbs et al.	OMI	13/13	PB-derived Cultured EPCs	RT	Effective	[79]
Assmus et al.	OMI	24/23	PB-derived Cultured EPCs	RCT	Ineffective	[80]
Boyle et al.	OMI	5/0	Gm-PB-CD34	NRT	NA	[81]
Losordo et al.	AP	18/6	Gm-PB-CD34	RT	Safe and feasible	[48]
Lara-Hernandez et al.	CLI	28/0	Gm-PB-CD34	Cohort	Effective	[82]
EPOCH-CLI	CLI	17/0	Gm-PB-CD34	Cohort	Effective	[50–52]
Kuroda et al.	NUF	4/0	Gm-PB-CD34	Cohort	Effective	Ongoing in Kobe, Japan

AMI, acute myocardial infarction; *OMI*, old myocardial infarction; *RMI*, recent myocardial infarction; *AP*, angina pectoris; *CLI*, critical limb ischemia; *NUF*, nonunion fracture; *PB*, peripheral blood; *BM*, bone marrow; *Gm*, G-CSF (granulocyte colony-stimulating factor) mobilized; *T/C*, treatment/control; *RT*, randomized trial; *NRT*, nonrandomized trial; *NA*, not available.

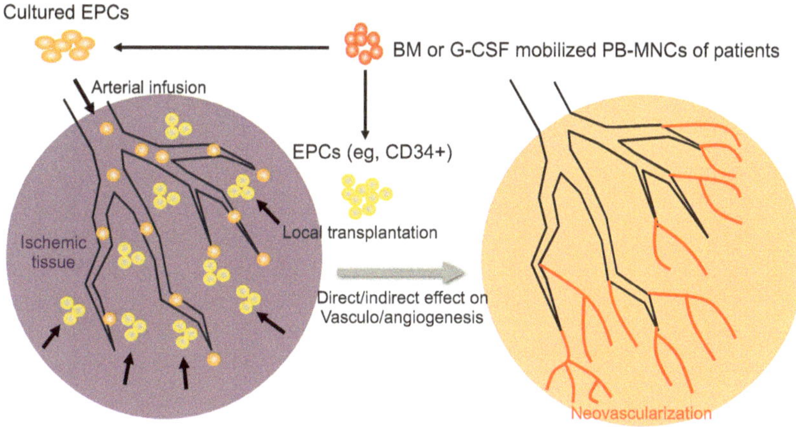

FIGURE 5.4 **Therapeutic angiogenesis/vasculogenesis via EPC transplantation. In clinical trials, both freshly isolated CD34+ cells from G-CSF mobilized mononuclear cells in peripheral blood (PB) of patients with chronic ischemic myocardial ischemia and cultured EPCs from BM or PB in patients with acute myocardial infarction have been used. EPCs lead to favorable outcomes regardless of the type of EPCs used.**

(TBPI), transcutaneous partial oxygen pressure ($TcPO_2$), total walking distance (TWD), pain-free walking distance (PFWD), Wang–Baker's pain rating scale, and ulcer size improved significantly after the transplantation of CD34+ cells. Because this was not a controlled randomized study, the possibility of a placebo effect after CD34+ cell transplantation needs to be evaluated in a large-scale

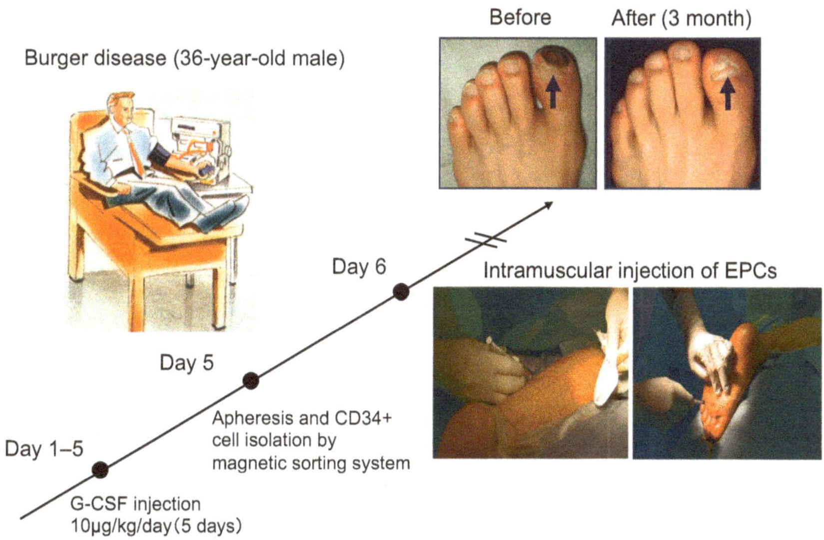

FIGURE 5.5 **Phase-I/II clinical trial regarding the intramuscular transplantation of autologous and G-CSF-mobilized CD34+ cells in patients with intractable critical limb ischemia (CLI).**

trial in the future. As for the evaluation of safety issues, neither death nor life-threatening adverse events were observed in this study, and no severe adverse events except for transient and expected mild to moderate ones could be observed as a result of the performed cell therapeutic approach.

The safety and efficacy of CD34+ cell therapy was sustained for up to 4 years after cell therapy [51]. Furthermore, our phase-II trial almost reproduced the clinical outcomes in the previous phase-I/IIa trial, indicating the safety, feasibility, and potential effectiveness of CD34+ cell transplantation for CLI patients [52]. Recently, in the ACT34-CLI (Autologous CD34+ Cell Therapy for Critical Limb Ischemia Investigator) study, a double-blind, randomized, placebo-controlled, phase-I/IIa pilot clinical trial, 28 patients with CLI due to ASO were randomized to receive intramuscular injection of 10^5 (low-dose, $n = 7$) or 10^6 (high-dose, $n = 9$) cells/kg of mobilized CD34+ cells or an equal volume of diluent. A favorable trend toward improvement of amputation-free survival rate was observed in the cell-treated groups, especially in the high-dose group, compared with control group at 6 and 12 months after treatment [53].

In addition to CD34, CD133 is a surface marker of early EPC phenotype. A recent clinical study by Burt et al. showed the safety and feasibility of autologous, GCSF-mobilized CD133+ cell implantation into lower extremity muscles of nine patients with CLI including a patient with Buerger's disease [54]. PB-MNCs were collected by leukapheresis after GCSF mobilization (10 μg/kg/day for 4–5 days), and CD133+ stem cells were selected using a magnetic separation system. There were no major complications from either leukapheresis or cell injection. The patient with Buerger's disease underwent the procedure twice. After the procedure, rest pain resolved rapidly by day 2, and seven of nine patients including a case of Buerger's disease were able to avoid limb amputation during the 1-year follow-up.

Although these studies were small-sized, nonrandomized trials, these initial results suggest the potential effectiveness of the purified EPC population in CLI patients.

As for the EPC therapy for coronary artery disease, Losordo et al. recently reported a phase-II, randomized, placebo-controlled, and dose-ranging clinical trial for 167 patients with refractory angina. Autologous CD34+ cells isolated from GCF-mobilized apheresis products were intramyocardially injected into ischemic myocardium under the guidance of NOGA endomyocardial mapping. Angina counts and changes in exercise time significantly improved in CD34+ cell group than placebo group after 6 and 12 months [55]. These promising outcomes also support the clinical usefulness of EPC transplantation for reduction of tissue ischemia.

These outcomes suggest the safety and feasibility of this cell-based therapy in patients with CLI.

Problems in EPC Transplantation

Our animal studies as well as the results of other groups suggest that heterologous EPC transplantation requires systemic injections of $0.5 \sim 2.0 \times 10^4$ human

EPCs/g body weight of the recipient animal to achieve a satisfactory improvement of hindlimb ischemia [2,40,44,56,57]. In general, cultured EPCs obtained from healthy human volunteers yield 5.0×10^6 cells per 100 mL of peripheral blood on day 7. On the basis of these data in human, a blood volume of as much as 12 L will be necessary to obtain a sufficient number of EPCs for the treatment of patients with critical hindlimb ischemia. Therefore, the background factors in clinical patients such as aging [58], diabetes [23,59], hypercholesterolemia [23], hypertension [23,60], and smoking [61,62] that may reduce the number and biological activity of circulating/BM EPCs represent possible major limitations for the success of primary EPC transplantations. In reality, most of the patients who are going to undergo EPC therapy for ischemic diseases have background diseases as described previously. Considering autologous EPC therapy, certain technical improvements that may help to overcome the shortcomings of EPCs should include: (1) local delivery of EPCs, (2) endogenous EPC mobilization, that is, cytokine/growth factor supplementation to promote BM-derived EPC mobilization [3,22], (3) enrichment procedures, that is, leukapheresis or BM aspiration, (4) enhancement of EPC functions by gene transduction, or (5) culture-expansion of EPCs from self-renewable primitive stem/progenitor cells isolated from BM or other sources. Unless the quality and quantity of autologous EPCs can be increased by the introduction of such technical improvements as mentioned previously, allogenic EPCs derived from umbilical cord blood or culture-expanded/generated EPCs from human ES/iPS cells [25,63], may serve as alternative sources for the supply of therapeutic active EPCs.

Future Strategies for EPC-Based Therapeutic Angiogenesis

Strategies that will recover potential EPC dysfunction and improve the bioactivity of these cells for the successful treatment of ischemic disorders should be considered, especially, in light of the current findings implicating that EPC function and mobilization may be impaired in certain diseases. One such strategy, the genetic modification and "enhancement" of EPCs with, for example, the targeted overexpression of proangiogenic growth factors in these cells, may enhance the angiogenic response and reactivate the bioactivity and/or extend the life span of EPCs.

In terms of increasing the quality of EPCs, we have shown that gene-modified EPCs could rescue impaired neovascularization in an animal model of limb ischemia [64]. Transplantation of heterologous EPCs transduced with adenovirus encoding human VEGF165 improved neovascularization and blood-flow recovery, reducing the limb necrosis and autoamputation rate in comparison with controls. The dose of EPCs needed to achieve limb salvage in these in vivo experiments was 30 times less than that required in the previous experiments involving unmodified EPCs [24]. Other investigators have also demonstrated the therapeutic efficacy of genetically engineered EPCs with a variety of targeted genes such as adrenomedullin (AM) [65], eNOS [66], tissue plasminogen activator (tPA) [67], and integrin-like kinase (ILK) [68] in animal models. Thus, genetic modification might overcome the potential problems associated with "less potent" patient EPCs and increase the therapeutic efficacy of such approaches, possibly, leading to the widespread use of these so-called "second generation EPC therapies." Combination of EPC cell based therapy with gene (ie, VEGF) therapy [69] or the combined use of proangiogenic, vascular stabilizing factors, that is, angiopoietin-1 and vasohibin-2 may also improve and overcome some of the current limitations experienced in the field. In addition, we have also recently succeeded to expand freshly isolated G-CSF mobilized PB-derived human CD34+ cells up to 20–50 times of their original cell number with growth factor/cytokine cocktail supplemented medium under serum-free conditions. Furthermore, these culture-expanded hCD34+ cells also exhibited higher therapeutic efficacy in vivo showing increased proangiogenic cytokine expressions in vitro compared to freshly isolated hCD34+ cells (unpublished data). This strategy might compensate the current disadvantages of applying dysfunctional EPCs for autologous cell transplantation therapy in ischemic diseases by increasing the quantity and quality of the applied EPCs.

Summary

Accumulating evidence suggests that BM-derived EPCs have the potential to promote postnatal vasculogenesis in adults, thus opening the way for possible clinical applications and the targeted cellular therapy of cardiovascular diseases. For a successful therapeutic EPC-based approach, the isolation and preparation of an optimal quality/quantity of EPCs is essential, making the resolution of certain still unresolved issues in the field a pressing prerequirement, such as (1) the development of better and more efficient EPC purification and expansion methods, (2) the improvement of administration and cellular application techniques, and (3) the "recovery" of the disease-based dysfunction and/or senescence of patient derived EPCs.

All these aforementioned aspects and awaited breakthroughs are undeniably also linked to and hampered by the lack of a clear and unambiguous definition of EPCs and the shear multitude of proposed EPC phenotypes, some of which we have tried to introduce and summarize earlier. A unified and generally accepted definition of EPCs, currently comprising a huge variety of cells used for animal studies or clinical applications, is allowing a detailed and meaningful molecular and/or functional characterization of these cells, and permitting subsequent proper interpretation of the observed preclinical and/or clinical phenotypes is unfortunately still missing. Surprisingly, the huge variety of applied "EPCs" ranging from HSC-related CD34/CD133 positive cells to utterly heterogeneous cell populations such as BM-MNCs seems to be still acceptable for the majority of "pragmatic" clinical investigators desperately searching for any "working" tools in their fight against cardiovascular diseases. The use of "easily accessible" cell populations such as BM/PB derived CD34+ cells will likely continue into the near future, especially with technical improvements regarding the isolation and application of these cells as well as the introduction of novel approaches of "pretreatment and modification" possibly further increasing the angiogenic properties of these cells. Other "easily accessible" cell types such as mesenchymal stem cells or "novel" subpopulations of MNCs such as CD31+ cells as well as ES/IPs-derived populations of patient-specific endothelial (progenitor) cells may also enter the arena of vascular therapy in the near future, especially after overcoming current technical limitations of proper generation and propagation of such cell populations.

The rather sobering results of many clinical trials assessing the efficacy and safety of EPCs for the treatment of vascular diseases should thus be taken as an indication that many of the still remaining basic questions regarding EPCs, such as the ultimate clarification and characterization of all phenotypical manifestations of EPCs, should be taken seriously and addressed before real breakthroughs in the use of this promising tool can be anticipated.

REFERENCES

[1] Asahara T, Murohara T, Sullivan A, Silver M, van der Zee R, Li T, et al. Isolation of putative progenitor endothelial cells for angiogenesis. Science 1997;275(5302):964–7.

[2] Asahara T, Masuda H, Takahashi T, Kalka C, Pastore C, Silver M, et al. Bone marrow origin of endothelial progenitor cells responsible for postnatal vasculogenesis in physiological and pathological neovascularization. Circ Res 1999;85(3):221–8.

[3] Asahara T, Takahashi T, Masuda H, Kalka C, Chen D, Iwaguro H, et al. VEGF contributes to postnatal neovascularization by mobilizing bone marrow-derived endothelial progenitor cells. EMBO J 1999;18(14):3964–72.

[4] Lyden D, Hattori K, Dias S, Costa C, Blaikie P, Butros L, et al. Impaired recruitment of bone-marrow-derived endothelial and hematopoietic precursor cells blocks tumor angiogenesis and growth. Nat Med 2001;7(11):1194–201.

[5] Beltrami AP, Barlucchi L, Torella D, Baker M, Limana F, Chimenti S, et al. Adult cardiac stem cells are multipotent and support myocardial regeneration. Cell 2003;114(6):763–76.

[6] Ii M, Nishimura H, Sekiguchi H, Kamei N, Yokoyama A, Horii M, et al. Concurrent vasculogenesis and neurogenesis from adult neural stem cells. Circ Res 2009;105(9):860–8.

[7] Kovacic JC, Boehm M. Resident vascular progenitor cells: an emerging role for non-terminally differentiated vessel-resident cells in vascular biology. Stem Cell Res 2009;2(1):2–15.

[8] Quirici N, Soligo D, Caneva L, Servida F, Bossolasco P, Deliliers GL. Differentiation and expansion of endothelial cells from human bone marrow CD133(+) cells. Br J Haematol 2001;115(1):186–94.

[9] Peichev M, Naiyer AJ, Pereira D, Zhu Z, Lane WJ, Williams M, et al. Expression of VEGFR-2 and AC133 by circulating human CD34(+) cells identifies a population of functional endothelial precursors. Blood 2000;95(3):952–8.

[10] Handgretinger R, Gordon PR, Leimig T, Chen X, Buhring HJ, Niethammer D, et al. Biology and plasticity of CD133+ hematopoietic stem cells. Ann NY Acad Sci 2003;996:141–51.

[11] Gehling UM, Ergun S, Schumacher U, Wagener C, Pantel K, Otte M, et al. In vitro differentiation of endothelial cells from AC133-positive progenitor cells. Blood 2000; 95(10):3106–12.

[12] Friedrich EB, Walenta K, Scharlau J, Nickenig G, Werner N. CD34-/CD133+/VEGFR-2+ endothelial progenitor cell subpopulation with potent vasoregenerative capacities. Circ Res 2006;98(3):e20–5.

[13] Eggermann J, Kliche S, Jarmy G, Hoffmann K, Mayr-Beyrle U, Debatin KM, et al. Endothelial progenitor cell culture and differentiation in vitro: a methodological comparison using human umbilical cord blood. Cardiovasc Res 2003;58(2):478–86.

[14] Patschan D, Krupincza K, Patschan S, Zhang Z, Hamby C, Goligorsky MS. Dynamics of mobilization and homing of endothelial progenitor cells after acute renal ischemia: modulation by ischemic preconditioning. Am J Physiol Renal Physiol 2006;291(1):F176–85.

[15] Hamada H, Kim MK, Iwakura A, Ii M, Thorne T, Qin G, et al. Estrogen receptors alpha and beta mediate contribution of bone marrow-derived endothelial progenitor cells to functional recovery after myocardial infarction. Circulation 2006;114(21):2261–70.

[16] Iwakura A, Luedemann C, Shastry S, Hanley A, Kearney M, Aikawa R, et al. Estrogen-mediated, endothelial nitric oxide synthase-dependent mobilization of bone marrow-derived endothelial progenitor cells contributes to reendothelialization after arterial injury. Circulation 2003;108(25):3115–21.

[17] Heeschen C, Aicher A, Lehmann R, Fichtlscherer S, Vasa M, Urbich C, et al. Erythropoietin is a potent physiologic stimulus for endothelial progenitor cell mobilization. Blood 2003;102(4):1340–6.

[18] Kwon SM, Eguchi M, Wada M, Iwami Y, Hozumi K, Iwaguro H, et al. Specific Jagged-1 signal from bone marrow microenvironment is required for endothelial progenitor cell development for neovascularization. Circulation 2008;118(2):157–65.

[19] Tanaka R, Wada M, Kwon SM, Masuda H, Carr J, Ito R, et al. The effects of flap ischemia on normal and diabetic progenitor cell function. Plast Reconstr Surg 2008;121(6):1929–42.

[20] Kamei N, Kwon SM, Alev C, Ishikawa M, Yokoyama A, Nakanishi K, et al. Lnk deletion reinforces the function of bone marrow progenitors in promoting neovascularization and astrogliosis following spinal cord injury. Stem Cells 2010;28(2):365–75.

[21] Dimmeler S, Aicher A, Vasa M, Mildner-Rihm C, Adler K, Tiemann M, et al. HMG-CoA reductase inhibitors (statins) increase endothelial progenitor cells via the PI 3-kinase/Akt pathway. J Clin Invest 2001;108(3):391–7.

[22] Takahashi T, Kalka C, Masuda H, Chen D, Silver M, Kearney M, et al. Ischemia- and cytokine-induced mobilization of bone marrow-derived endothelial progenitor cells for neovascularization. Nat Med 1999;5(4):434–8.

[23] Vasa M, Fichtlscherer S, Aicher A, Adler K, Urbich C, Martin H, et al. Number and migratory activity of circulating endothelial progenitor cells inversely correlate with risk factors for coronary artery disease. Circ Res 2001;89(1):E1–7.

[24] Kalka C, Tehrani H, Laudenberg B, Vale PR, Isner JM, Asahara T, et al. VEGF gene transfer mobilizes endothelial progenitor cells in patients with inoperable coronary disease. Ann Thorac Surg 2000;70(3):829–34.

[25] Murohara T, Ikeda H, Duan J, Shintani S, Sasaki K, Eguchi H, et al. Transplanted cord blood-derived endothelial precursor cells augment postnatal neovascularization. J Clin Invest 2000;105(11):1527–36.

[26] Sharpe EE 3rd, Teleron AA, Li B, Price J, Sands MS, Alford K, et al. The origin and in vivo significance of murine and human culture-expanded endothelial progenitor cells. Am J Pathol 2006;168(5):1710–21.

[27] Timmermans F, Plum J, Yoder MC, Ingram DA, Vandekerckhove B, Case J. Endothelial progenitor cells: identity defined? J Cell Mol Med 2009;13(1):87–102.

[28] Gulati R, Jevremovic D, Peterson TE, Chatterjee S, Shah V, Vile RG, et al. Diverse origin and function of cells with endothelial phenotype obtained from adult human blood. Circ Res 2003;93(11):1023–5.

[29] Hur J, Yang HM, Yoon CH, Lee CS, Park KW, Kim JH, et al. Identification of a novel role of T cells in postnatal vasculogenesis: characterization of endothelial progenitor cell colonies. Circulation 2007;116(15):1671–82.

[30] Rehman J, Li J, Orschell CM, March KL. Peripheral blood "endothelial progenitor cells" are derived from monocyte/macrophages and secrete angiogenic growth factors. Circulation 2003;107(8):1164–9.

[31] Shepherd RM, Capoccia BJ, Devine SM, Dipersio J, Trinkaus KM, Ingram D, et al. Angiogenic cells can be rapidly mobilized and efficiently harvested from the blood following treatment with AMD3100. Blood 2006;108(12):3662–7.

[32] Folkman J, Shing Y. Angiogenesis. Journal of Biological Chemistry 1992;267:10931–4.

[33] Masuda H, Kalka C, Takahashi T, Yoshida M, Wada M, Kobori M, et al. Estrogen-mediated endothelial progenitor cell biology and kinetics for physiological postnatal vasculogenesis. Circ Res 2007;101(6):598–606.

[34] Bauer SM, Goldstein LJ, Bauer RJ, Chen H, Putt M, Velazquez OC. The bone marrow-derived endothelial progenitor cell response is impaired in delayed wound healing from ischemia. J Vasc Surg 2006;43(1):134–41.

[35] Ii M, Nishimura H, Iwakura A, Wecker A, Eaton E, Asahara T, et al. Endothelial progenitor cells are rapidly recruited to myocardium and mediate protective effect of ischemic preconditioning via "imported" nitric oxide synthase activity. Circulation 2005;111(9):1114–20.

[36] Iwakura A, Shastry S, Luedemann C, Hamada H, Kawamoto A, Kishore R, et al. Estradiol enhances recovery after myocardial infarction by augmenting incorporation of bone marrow-derived endothelial progenitor cells into sites of ischemia-induced neovascularization via endothelial nitric oxide synthase-mediated activation of matrix metalloproteinase-9. Circulation 2006;113(12):1605–14.

[37] Murayama T, Tepper OM, Silver M, Ma H, Losordo DW, Isner JM, et al. Determination of bone marrow-derived endothelial progenitor cell significance in angiogenic growth factor-induced neovascularization in vivo. Exp Hematol 2002;30(8):967–72.

[38] Tamaki T, Akatsuka A, Ando K, Nakamura Y, Matsuzawa H, Hotta T, et al. Identification of myogenic-endothelial progenitor cells in the interstitial spaces of skeletal muscle. J Cell Biol 2002;157(4):571–7.

[39] Miyamoto Y, Suyama T, Yashita T, Akimaru H, Kurata H. Bone marrow subpopulations contain distinct types of endothelial progenitor cells and angiogenic cytokine-producing cells. J Mol Cell Cardiol 2007;43(5):627–35.

[40] Kawamoto A, Gwon HC, Iwaguro H, Yamaguchi JI, Uchida S, Masuda H, et al. Therapeutic potential of ex vivo expanded endothelial progenitor cells for myocardial ischemia. Circulation 2001;103(5):634–7.

[41] Matsumoto T, Kawamoto A, Kuroda R, Ishikawa M, Mifune Y, Iwasaki H, et al. Therapeutic potential of vasculogenesis and osteogenesis promoted by peripheral blood CD34-positive cells for functional bone healing. Am J Pathol 2006;169(4):1440–57.

[42] Schatteman GC, Hanlon HD, Jiao C, Dodds SG, Christy BA. Blood-derived angioblasts accelerate blood-flow restoration in diabetic mice. J Clin Invest 2000;106(4):571–8.

[43] Kocher AA, Schuster MD, Szabolcs MJ, Takuma S, Burkhoff D, Wang J, et al. Neovascularization of ischemic myocardium by human bone-marrow-derived angioblasts prevents cardiomyocyte apoptosis, reduces remodeling and improves cardiac function. Nat Med 2001;7(4):430–6.

[44] Iwasaki H, Kawamoto A, Ishikawa M, Oyamada A, Nakamori S, Nishimura H, et al. Dose-dependent contribution of CD34-positive cell transplantation to concurrent vasculogenesis and cardiomyogenesis for functional regenerative recovery after myocardial infarction. Circulation 2006;113(10):1311–25.
[45] Asahara T, Kawamoto A. Endothelial progenitor cells for postnatal vasculogenesis. Am J Physiol Cell Physiol 2004;287(3):C572–9.
[46] Goldberg JL, Laughlin MJ. UC blood hematopoietic stem cells and therapeutic angiogenesis. Cytotherapy 2007;9(1):4–13.
[47] Losordo DW, Kishore R. A big promise from the very small identification of circulating embryonic stem-like pluripotent cells in patients with acute myocardial infarction. J Am Coll Cardiol 2009;53(1):10–2.
[48] Losordo DW, Schatz RA, White CJ, Udelson JE, Veereshwarayya V, Durgin M, et al. Intramyocardial transplantation of autologous CD34+ stem cells for intractable angina: a phase I/IIa double-blind, randomized controlled trial. Circulation 2007;115(25):3165–72.
[49] Jujo K, Ii M, Losordo DW. Endothelial progenitor cells in neovascularization of infarcted myocardium. J Mol Cell Cardiol 2008;45(4):530–44.
[50] Kawamoto A, Katayama M, Handa N, Kinoshita M, Takano H, Horii M, et al. Intramuscular transplantation of G-CSF-mobilized CD34(+) cells in patients with critical limb ischemia: a phase I/IIa, multicenter, single-blinded, dose-escalation clinical trial. Stem Cells 2009;27(11):2857–64.
[51] Kinoshita M, Fujita Y, Katayama M, Baba R, Shibakawa M, Yoshikawa K, et al. Long-term clinical outcome after intramuscular transplantation of granulocyte colony stimulating factor-mobilized CD34 positive cells in patients with critical limb ischemia. Atherosclerosis 2012;224(2):440–5.
[52] Fujita Y, Kinoshita M, Furukawa Y, Nagano T, Hashimoto H, Hirami Y, et al. Phase II clinical trial of CD34+ cell therapy to explore endpoint selection and timing in patients with critical limb ischemia. Circ J 2014;78(2):490–501.
[53] Losordo DW, Vale PR, Hendel RC, Milliken CE, Fortuin FD, Cummings N, et al. Phase 1/2 placebo-controlled, double-blind, dose-escalating trial of myocardial vascular endothelial growth factor 2 gene transfer by catheter delivery in patients with chronic myocardial ischemia. Circulation 2002;105(17):2012–8.
[54] Burt RK, Testori A, Oyama Y, Rodriguez HE, Yaung K, Villa M, et al. Autologous peripheral blood CD133+ cell implantation for limb salvage in patients with critical limb ischemia. Bone Marrow Transplant 2010;45(1):111–6.
[55] Losordo DW, Henry TD, Davidson C, Sup Lee J, Costa MA, Bass T, et al. Intramyocardial, autologous CD34+ cell therapy for refractory angina. Circ Res 2011;109(4):428–36.
[56] Kalka C, Masuda H, Takahashi T, Kalka-Moll WM, Silver M, Kearney M, et al. Transplantation of ex vivo expanded endothelial progenitor cells for therapeutic neovascularization. Proc Natl Acad Sci USA 2000;97(7):3422–7.
[57] Hung HS, Shyu WC, Tsai CH, Hsu SH, Lin SZ. Transplantation of endothelial progenitor cells as therapeutics for cardiovascular diseases. Cell Transplant 2009;18(9):1003–12.
[58] Heiss C, Keymel S, Niesler U, Ziemann J, Kelm M, Kalka C. Impaired progenitor cell activity in age-related endothelial dysfunction. J Am Coll Cardiol 2005;45(9):1441–8.
[59] Ii M, Takenaka H, Asai J, Ibusuki K, Mizukami Y, Maruyama K, et al. Endothelial progenitor thrombospondin-1 mediates diabetes-induced delay in reendothelialization following arterial injury. Circ Res 2006;98(5):697–704.
[60] Imanishi T, Moriwaki C, Hano T, Nishio I. Endothelial progenitor cell senescence is accelerated in both experimental hypertensive rats and patients with essential hypertension. J Hypertens 2005;23(10):1831–7.

[61] Kondo T, Hayashi M, Takeshita K, Numaguchi Y, Kobayashi K, Iino S, et al. Smoking cessation rapidly increases circulating progenitor cells in peripheral blood in chronic smokers. Arterioscler Thromb Vasc Biol 2004;24(8):1442–7.
[62] Michaud SE, Dussault S, Haddad P, Groleau J, Rivard A. Circulating endothelial progenitor cells from healthy smokers exhibit impaired functional activities. Atherosclerosis 2006;187(2):423–32.
[63] Levenberg S, Golub JS, Amit M, Itskovitz-Eldor J, Langer R. Endothelial cells derived from human embryonic stem cells. Proc Natl Acad Sci USA 2002;99(7):4391–6.
[64] Iwaguro H, Yamaguchi J, Kalka C, Murasawa S, Masuda H, Hayashi S, et al. Endothelial progenitor cell vascular endothelial growth factor gene transfer for vascular regeneration. Circulation 2002;105(6):732–8.
[65] Nagaya N, Kangawa K, Kanda M, Uematsu M, Horio T, Fukuyama N, et al. Hybrid cell-gene therapy for pulmonary hypertension based on phagocytosing action of endothelial progenitor cells. Circulation 2003;108(7):889–95.
[66] Kong D, Melo LG, Mangi AA, Zhang L, Lopez-Ilasaca M, Perrella MA, et al. Enhanced inhibition of neointimal hyperplasia by genetically engineered endothelial progenitor cells. Circulation 2004;109(14):1769–75.
[67] Griese DP, Achatz S, Batzlsperger CA, Strauch UG, Grumbeck B, Weil J, et al. Vascular gene delivery of anticoagulants by transplantation of retrovirally-transduced endothelial progenitor cells. Cardiovasc Res 2003;58(2):469–77.
[68] Cho HJ, Youn SW, Cheon SI, Kim TY, Hur J, Zhang SY, et al. Regulation of endothelial cell and endothelial progenitor cell survival and vasculogenesis by integrin-linked kinase. Arterioscler Thromb Vasc Biol 2005;25(6):1154–60.
[69] Kawamoto A, Murayama T, Kusano K, Ii M, Tkebuchava T, Shintani S, et al. Synergistic effect of bone marrow mobilization and vascular endothelial growth factor-2 gene therapy in myocardial ischemia. Circulation 2004;110(11):1398–405.
[70] Schachinger V, Assmus B, Britten MB, Honold J, Lehmann R, Teupe C, et al. Transplantation of progenitor cells and regeneration enhancement in acute myocardial infarction: final one-year results of the TOPCARE-AMI Trial. J Am Coll Cardiol 2004;44(8):1690–9.
[71] Bartunek J, Vanderheyden M, Vandekerckhove B, Mansour S, De Bruyne B, De Bondt P, et al. Intracoronary injection of CD133-positive enriched bone marrow progenitor cells promotes cardiac recovery after recent myocardial infarction: feasibility and safety. Circulation 2005;112(9 Suppl):I178–83.
[72] Ii M, Losordo DW. Statins and the endothelium. Vascul Pharmacol 2007;46(1):1–9.
[73] Tatsumi T, Ashihara E, Yasui T, Matsunaga S, Kido A, Sasada Y, et al. Intracoronary transplantation of non-expanded peripheral blood-derived mononuclear cells promotes improvement of cardiac function in patients with acute myocardial infarction. Circ J 2007;71(8):1199–207.
[74] Dobert N, Britten M, Assmus B, Berner U, Menzel C, Lehmann R, et al. Transplantation of progenitor cells after reperfused acute myocardial infarction: evaluation of perfusion and myocardial viability with FDG-PET and thallium SPECT. Eur J Nucl Med Mol Imag 2004;31(8):1146–51.
[75] Stamm C, Westphal B, Kleine HD, Petzsch M, Kittner C, Klinge H, et al. Autologous bone-marrow stem-cell transplantation for myocardial regeneration. Lancet 2003;361(9351):45–6.
[76] Stamm C, Kleine HD, Choi YH, Dunkelmann S, Lauffs JA, Lorenzen B, et al. Intramyocardial delivery of CD133+ bone marrow cells and coronary artery bypass grafting for chronic ischemic heart disease: safety and efficacy studies. J Thorac Cardiovasc Surg 2007;133(3):717–25.
[77] Ahmadi H, Baharvand H, Ashtiani SK, Soleimani M, Sadeghian H, Ardekani JM, et al. Safety analysis and improved cardiac function following local autologous transplantation

of CD133(+) enriched bone marrow cells after myocardial infarction. Curr Neurovasc Res 2007;4(3):153–60.
[78] Balogh L, Czuriga I, Hunyadi J, Galuska L, Kristof E, Edes I. Effects of autologous bone marrow derived CD34+ stem cells on the left ventricular function following myocardial infarction. Orv Hetil 2007;148(6):243–9.
[79] Erbs S, Linke A, Adams V, Lenk K, Thiele H, Diederich KW, et al. Transplantation of blood-derived progenitor cells after recanalization of chronic coronary artery occlusion: first randomized and placebo-controlled study. Circ Res 2005;97(8):756–62.
[80] Assmus B, Honold J, Schachinger V, Britten MB, Fischer-Rasokat U, Lehmann R, et al. Transcoronary transplantation of progenitor cells after myocardial infarction. N Engl J Med 2006;355(12):1222–32.
[81] Kocher AA, Schuster MD, Bonaros N, Lietz K, Xiang G, Martens TP, et al. Myocardial homing and neovascularization by human bone marrow angioblasts is regulated by IL-8/Gro CXC chemokines. J Mol Cell Cardiol 2006;40(4):455–64.
[82] Lara-Hernandez R, Lozano-Vilardell P, Blanes P, Torreguitart-Mirada N, Galmes A, Besalduch J. Safety and efficacy of therapeutic angiogenesis as a novel treatment in patients with critical limb ischemia. Ann Vasc Surg 2010;24(2):287–94.

Chapter 6

Mature Cell Activation

K.S. Telukuntla, MD, M.Y. Flugelman, MD, E.R. Mohler III, MD
Perelman School of Medicine at the University of Pennsylvania, Division of Cardiovascular Medicine, Department of Medicine, Philadelphia, PA, United States

Cell therapy continues to be a promising approach to develop novel therapeutic interventions for the treatment of peripheral artery disease (PAD). Preclinical and clinical trials have utilized various single cell lines or combinatorial approaches with multiple cell types [1,2]. Several trials have demonstrated the role of antigen-specific cells, whereas others have demonstrated that the administration of the milieu of cytokines including vascular endothelial growth factor (VEGF), fibroblast growth factor, and hypoxia-inducible factor 1-alpha can augment the desired arteriogenesis. More importantly, only two studies have proposed the concept of ex vivo genetic modification to enhance cell therapy in clinical trials. The first was the phase-I Safety, Dose Escalating Study of MultiGeneAngio (MGA) in Patients with Peripheral Arterial Disease (NCT00390767) and the second study titled Safety Study of MGA in Patients with Chronic Critical Limb Ischemia (NCT00956332) assessed the safety profile of MGA in 23 patients with chronic critical limb ischemia [3,4]. This chapter will focus on this concept of mature cell activation and its potential application in the field of PAD.

Ex vivo genetic modification is the process of removing cells from a patient and subsequent DNA transduction using retroviral vectors to upregulate or downregulate target genes. The field of oncology has tried to use this approach to develop cancer therapies as early as the 1980s when Zelig Eshhar and Steven Rosenberg constructed the first chimeric antigen receptor (CAR) T- cells [5]. Most recently, this technique has been successfully employed in the novel chimeric antigen receptor-modified T cells (CART-19) therapies for acute lymphoblastic leukemia and chronic lymphocytic leukemia [6,7]. CART-19 therapy was developed by Dr Carl June and his team at the University of Pennsylvania, Perelman School of Medicine, and its affiliated Children's Hospital of Philadelphia. As of July 2014, CART-19 therapy was granted Breakthrough Therapy designation by the US Food and Drug Administration for treatment of both relapsed and refractory acute lymphoblastic leukemia (ALL) in adults and children [8].

Regenerative Medicine for Peripheral Artery Disease. http://dx.doi.org/10.1016/B978-0-12-801344-1.00006-1

The ex vivo genetic modification approach was also recently employed by researchers in China who were studying vascular endothelial injury in the setting of postthrombotic syndrome (PTS) [9]. Tang et al. constructed rat models with inferior vena cava thrombosis by applying ferric chloride to simulate PTS pathology. Adenovirus transfection was utilized to upregulate VEGF165 in the endothelial progenitor cells (EPCs). Subsequent transplantation of the EPCs into the injured vascular endothelium led to a significantly faster repair of the postthrombotic tunica intima layer. Although this study did not delve into the exact mechanisms of action to explain the findings, it has been previously reported that VEGF overexpression can promote angiogenesis and enable vessel restoration [10].

VEGF overexpression was also utilized as part of the Multi-gene Cell Therapy Study (NCT00390767) [4]. This is a nonrandomized and unblinded phase-I trial to assess the safety of autologous venous endothelial and smooth muscle cells called MultiGeneAngio (MGA) which is a novel cell-based therapy with ex vivo modification to express growth factors implicated in angiogenesis. Each of the 12 patients received transduced autologous venous smooth muscle cells that express vascular endothelial growth factor (VEGF165) and endothelial cells that express Angiopoietin-1 (Ang-1).

All 12 patients were male with a median age of 60 ± 5. All had a history of PAD confirmed by ankle–brachial index (ABI) <0.90 and exercise treadmill protocol that confirmed symptoms of claudication. Comorbidities included diabetes mellitus (25%), hyperlipidemia (92%), hypertension (92%), coronary artery disease (75%), and smoking history (92%). In addition to other exclusion criteria, patients with critical limb ischemia that produced rest pain, lower extremity arterial ulcers, or gangrene were excluded.

Cells were first isolated from the patient's cephalic or basilic veins using techniques detailed in the manuscript and then used to engineer the MGA suspension. The endothelial and smooth muscle cells were transduced with retroviral vectors that encode Ang-1 and VEGF-165, respectively. Both of these proteins have been implicated in angiogenesis. Coexpression is required to ensure vessel wall integrity. Ang-1 is known to play a critical role in vessel wall maturation and reducing vascular permeability whereas upregulation of VEGF would lead to permeable vessels. Use of fully differentiated, somatic vascular cells genetically engineered to express VEGF and Ang-1 was shown to produce arteriogenesis in vitro and in vivo [11]. Once MGA suspension was manufactured, it was delivered via an intraarterial approach. The untreated common femoral artery was cannulated and a catheter was used to cross over to the location of the occlusion which was either in the superficial or common femoral artery. After angiograms were performed, the MGA suspension was injected and the catheter and sheath were removed with proper hemostasis.

The 12 subjects were monitored throughout the duration of the study by graded treadmill testing at the time of screening, day 30, day 90, day 180, and day 365. The peak walking time and mean claudication onset time increased

($p < 0.05$) during the follow-up interval. In regards to the safety profile of the MGA suspension and intraarterial delivery, there were four serious adverse events documented. One of the patients had a history of left ventricle thrombus and thromboembolic episode suffered a transient ischemic attack 7 months after receiving MGA therapy. The second patient experienced an obstructive dissection of the contralateral iliac artery 10 days after the catheterization. The principal investigators of this trial thought this adverse event was related to the MGA treatment catheterization procedure. The third patient suffered from acute leg ischemia secondary to an occluding thrombus in the iliac artery 6 months after the procedure which was thought to be related to subtherapeutic INRs in the setting of a mechanical aortic valve. The fourth patient experienced a myocardial infarction 6 months after the procedure and required coronary artery bypass grafts.

This was the first clinical trial utilizing ex vivo modification of mature cells to promote angiogenesis in patients with PAD. This phase-I trial demonstrated the safety profile of MGA, but the small cohort of patients and the nonrandomized approach make it difficult to assess efficacy. Confirmation of safety and feasibility of such therapy was received in the second phase-I trial conducted in patients with critical limb ischemia. The concept of cell activation has been promising and further large-scale randomized clinical trials are needed to demonstrate efficacy of this approach.

DISCLOSURES

ERM and KST have no disclosures. MYF is the Founder of MGVS Ltd that financed the studies described in this manuscript.

REFERENCES

[1] Cooke JP, Losordo DW. Modulating the vascular response to limb ischemia: angiogenic and cell therapies. Circ Res 2015;116(9):1561–78.

[2] Ouma GO, Zafrir B, Mohler ER, Flugelman MY. Therapeutic angiogenesis in critical limb ischemia. Angiology 2013;64(6):466–80.

[3] MultiGene Vascular Systems Ltd. Safety study of MultiGeneAngio in patients with chronic critical limb ischemia (NCT00956332); 2015. Available from: https://www.clinicaltrials.gov/ct2/show/NCT00956332?term=NCT00956332&rank=1

[4] Grossman PM, Mohler ER, Roessler BJ, Wilensky RL, Levine BL, Woo EY, et al. Phase I study of multi-gene cell therapy in patients with peripheral artery disease. Vasc Med 2015; 21(1):21–32.

[5] Gross G, Waks T, Eshhar Z. Expression of immunoglobulin-T-cell receptor chimeric molecules as functional receptors with antibody-type specificity. Proc Natl Acad Sci USA 1989;86:10024.

[6] Grupp SA, Kalos M, Barrett D, Aplenc R, Porter DL, Rheingold SR, et al. Chimeric antigen receptor–modified T cells for acute lymphoid leukemia. N Engl J Med 2013; 368(16): 1509–1518.

[7] Porter DL, Levine BL, Kalos M, Bagg A, June CH. Chimeric antigen receptor–modified T cells in chronic lymphoid leukemia. N Engl J Med 2011;2016;365(8):725–733.

[8] Gill S, June CH. Going viral: chimeric antigen receptor T-cell therapy for hematological malignancies. Immunol Rev 2015;263(1):68–89.
[9] Tang J, Meng Q, Cai Z, Li X. Transplantation of VEGFl65-overexpressing vascular endothelial progenitor cells relieves endothelial injury after deep vein thrombectomy. Thromb Res 2016;137:41–5.
[10] Meng Q, Li X, Yu X, Lei F, Jiang KLC. Transplantation of VEGF165-gene-transfected endothelial progenitor cells in the treatment of chronic venous thrombosis in rats. Chinese Med J 2010;123:471.
[11] Gluzman Z, Koren B, Preis M, Cohen T, Tsaba A, Cosset F, et al. Endothelial cells are activated by angiopoeitin-1 gene transfer and produce coordinated sprouting in vitro and arteriogenesis in vivo. Biochem Biophys Res Commun 2007;359(2):263–8.

Chapter 7

Imaging for Regenerative Therapy for PAD

C.M. Kramer, MD, M. Yadava, MD, J.R. Lindner, MD

Departments of Medicine, Radiology and Medical Imaging, and the Cardiovascular Imaging Center, University of Virginia Health System, Charlottesville, VA and the Knight Cardiovascular Institute, Oregon Health & Science University, Portland, OR, United States

INTRODUCTION

Over the past few decades, angiography has been the mainstay of imaging of the lower extremity vasculature, first with digital subtraction angiography (DSA) and, more recently, with magnetic resonance angiography (MRA) and computed tomographic angiography (CTA). Angiographic techniques are excellent at assessing patency and status of the larger arteries within the lower extremity in patients with peripheral artery disease (PAD), but are not quantitative and are unable to assess smaller vessels, including collaterals, or perfusion at the tissue level. Doppler ultrasound provides information on the degree of stenosis of large vessels of the lower limb but again does not assess tissue perfusion. The ability to image smaller vessels and measure tissue perfusion is an unmet clinical need in the evaluation of patients with PAD who are candidates for regeneration therapy with stem cells or other angiogenic therapies. Potential improvements with these therapies are more likely to be at the microvascular level, which cannot be assessed by traditional angiography or by conventional pressure-based methods [eg, ankle–brachial index (ABI)] for assessing PAD severity. In this regard, newer techniques such as MRI perfusion imaging, PET, single photon emission tomography radionuclide imaging (RNI), and CEU are in various stages of development for this important use. To date, there have been few studies using these techniques as endpoints in trials of regenerative therapies. This chapter reviews these potential endpoints for use in future studies of novel approaches to PAD.

MAGNETIC RESONANCE IMAGING AND SPECTROSCOPY

In the past decade, major advances have been made in the ability to measure tissue perfusion and energetics in the leg muscle of patients with PAD. Skeletal muscle resting perfusion is extremely low and thus very difficult to measure.

Regenerative Medicine for Peripheral Artery Disease. http://dx.doi.org/10.1016/B978-0-12-801344-1.00007-3

Thus, testing of perfusion and energetics requires a physiological challenge that normally creates hyperemia. This can be done with exercise with an MR-compatible ergometer or cuff occlusion. During a cuff occlusion paradigm, a blood pressure cuff is inflated in the proximal thigh to at least 50 mmHg above the individual's systolic blood pressure causing tissue ischemia and hypoxia. The cuff is kept inflated for 5 min and then rapidly deflated. Following deflation there is generalized reactive hyperemia.

Skeletal Muscle Perfusion

The primary MR methods to assess skeletal muscle perfusion are first-pass contrast enhanced (CE-MRI) and arterial spin labeling (ASL) MRI. Both techniques provide spatially and temporally resolved measures of skeletal muscle perfusion. Both techniques can be used with either exercise or cuff-occlusion.

First-pass CE-MRI uses a T1-weighted sequence to visualize contrast-enhanced blood flow into tissue over time. It can be used to calculate skeletal muscle perfusion both semiquantitatively and fully quantitatively on a mL/100 g/min basis using a two-compartment model which has been validated in animal studies of myocardial blood flow using microspheres as a reference technique [1,2]. Thompson et al. used a modified first-pass CE-MRI method with cuff-occlusion [3]. Contrast was administered immediately after cuff inflation, both producing ischemia and allowing contrast to equilibrate in the arterial blood pool, while excluding it from the lower limb. With cuff release, a true step-input of contrast was produced that coincided with hyperemic blood flow. Although no direct validation or limits of agreement analysis were done and only one PAD patient was studied, the experiments yielded flow rates comparable to other techniques. This method is limited to a cuff occlusion approach since contrast has to equilibrate in the arterial blood pool prior to hyperemia.

A semiquantitative method using first-pass CE-MRI is to measure a perfusion index (PI), defined as the slope of the tissue time–intensity curve (TF) divided by the slope of the arterial time–intensity curve (AIF) from the feeding artery [4] (Fig. 7.1). In a study of 11 PAD patients and 22 normal volunteers, PI at peak exercise was significantly lower in PAD patients than normals. The difference remained significant even in a group of normal volunteers who matched the PAD patient's lower workload. The method proved effective in differentiating PAD patients from normal volunteers with an area under the receiver operating characteristic (ROC) curve of 0.88 and 0.95 when including all normal volunteers and only volunteers who performed maximum workload, respectively. Interobserver agreement was high, with an intraclass correlation coefficient (ICC) of 0.91. In a follow-up study, PI was shown to be moderately reproducible when studies were performed on separate days with an ICC of 0.60 [5]. The latter study showed that perfusion reserve, defined as the exercise TF/rest TF, was preserved in PAD and not useful to differentiate

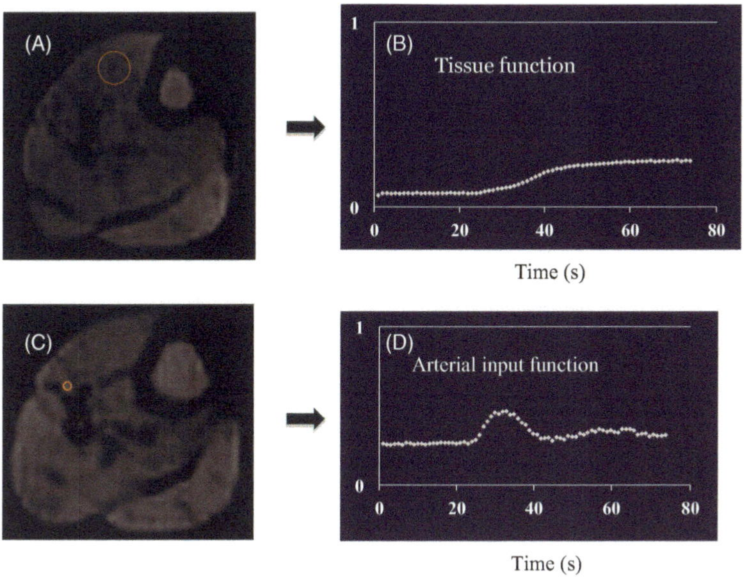

FIGURE 7.1 (A) Tissue slice from contrast-enhanced cross-sectional image of the calf from a PAD patient. Large ROI has been placed in the anterior tibialis to measure a signal intensity time curve for the tissue function shown at (B). (C) Arterial input slice taken superior to the tissue slice shown previously with an ROI placed in the feeding tibial artery to measure a signal intensity time curve for the arterial input as shown at (D).

PAD patients from normal volunteers, due to extremely low rest values in both patients and volunteers.

ASL is a contrast-free method that magnetically labels protons in arterial blood which then create changes in signal intensity within the imaging slice as blood flows into the slice. ASL provides flow measurements on a mL/100g/min basis and has been validated against venous occlusion plethysmography [6]. In a study of 40 PAD patients and 17 age-matched controls using continuous ASL and cuff occlusion, Wu et al. found a direct correlation between PAD severity, peak hyperemic flow, and time to peak (TTP) hyperemic flow [7] (Fig. 7.2). The TTP hyperemic flow was affected with early changes in ankle–brachial index (ABI), whereas peak hyperemic flow was preserved until the more advanced stages of the disease. Pollak et al. studied the performance of pulsed ASL using exercise in 15 PAD patients and 15 normal volunteers [8]. Mean peak exercise flow was significantly greater in normal volunteers than PAD patients (Fig. 7.3). Similar to contrast-enhanced measures[4], the difference remained significant when a predetermined group of normal volunteers matched PAD patients' workload. Twelve studies were repeated in 7 PAD patients and 5 normal volunteers. The ICC was 0.87 and 0.96 for repeated studies and interobserver reproducibility, respectively, and thus better than the semiquantitative contrast-enhanced methods discussed previously.

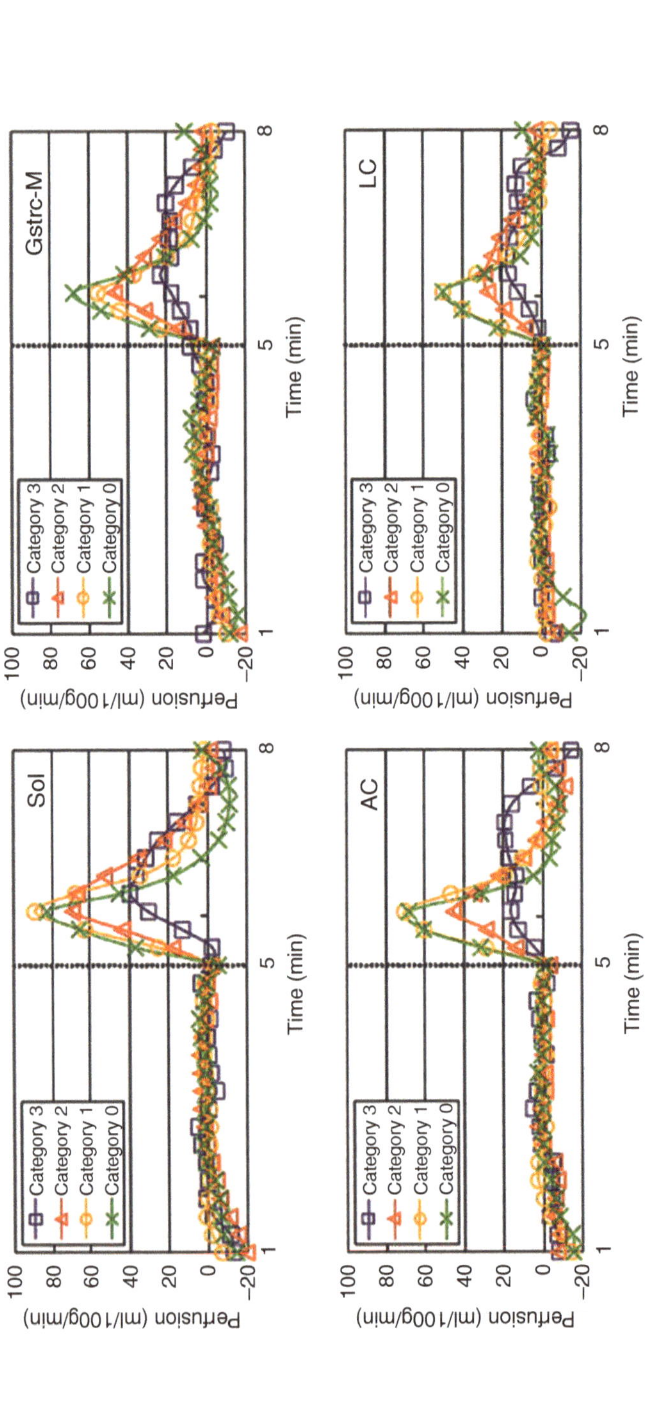

FIGURE 7.2 **ASL perfusion time curves for four different muscle groups (soleus, gastrocnemius, anterior compartment, lateral compartment) for four different categories of ABI's with third category representing the lowest ABI's and the shallowest perfusion time curves.** *(Reproduced with permission from Ref. [7].)*

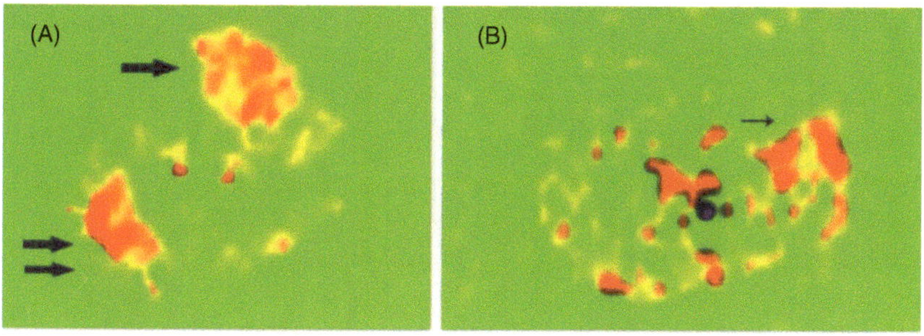

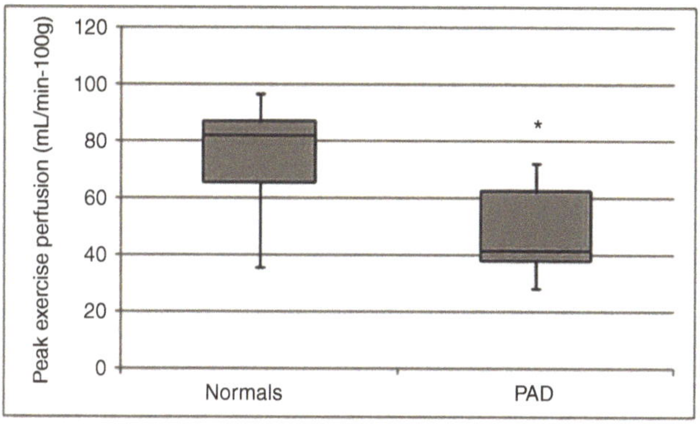

FIGURE 7.3 **Images A and B show postexercise ASL calf-muscle perfusion in a normal volunteer (A) and PAD subject (B).** Shown is an axial image of the calf belonging to a normal volunteer (A) with increased muscle blood flow seen in red for both the anterior tibialis (*arrow*) and gastrocnemius muscles (*double arrow*). For the PAD subject (B) the axial image shows increase calf muscle blood flow in the gastrocneumius (*thin arrow*). The following *box plot* shows median peak exercise calf muscle perfusion in normals and PAD subjects. The *down whisker* represents the first quartile minus the minimum value and up whisker represents the maximum minus the third quartile. * $p < 0.001$ versus normals. *(Reproduced with permission from Ref. [8].)*

Skeletal Muscle Deoxygenation

Blood oxygen level dependent (BOLD) MRI is sensitive to the paramagnetic concentration of deoxyhemoglobin which results in a T2* signal loss. Both exercise and cuff-occlusion can be used to study the BOLD signal in PAD patients. During cuff-occlusion there is T2* signal loss and during reactive hyperemia or exercise, there is T2* signal gain due to increased oxyhemoglobin content [9]. Thus, changes in BOLD signal offer an indirect measure of tissue perfusion and have been correlated to skeletal muscle perfusion by relaxometry [10] and ASL MRI [11].

Using cuff occlusion, Lederman et. al. measured the maximum change in T2* ($\Delta T2^*_{max}$) signal and the TTP maximal T2* signal in the calf of PAD patients and age-matched controls [12] (Fig. 7.4). They found that the $\Delta T2^*_{max}$ was significantly lower and TTP significantly longer in PAD patients compared

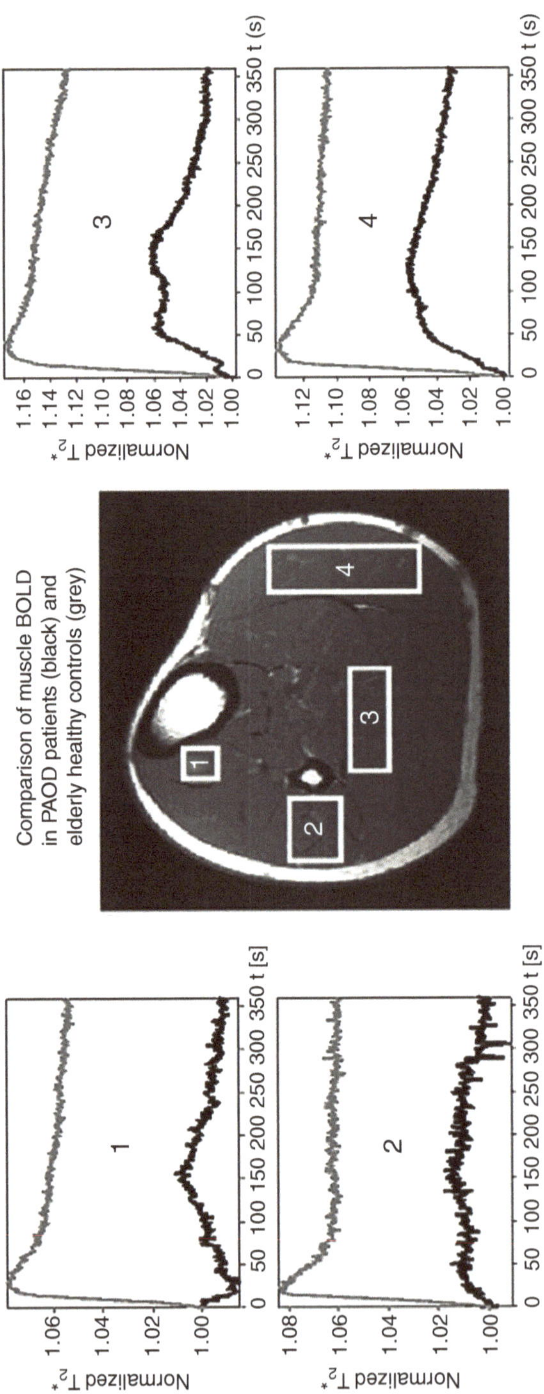

FIGURE 7.4 Normalized T2* time course (BOLD response) during 360 s of reactive hyperemia in PAD patients (*n* = 17; black) and age-matched healthy volunteers (*n* = 11; gray) for individual calf muscles. Representative regions of interest for anterior tibialis (1), peroneal (2), soleus (3) and medial gastrocnemius (4) muscles are overlaid on corresponding T1-weighted image (*middle panel*). *(Reproduced with permission from Ref. [12].)*

to controls. There was a good correlation between TTP and the ABI. With one exception, all PAD patients with ABI < 1 had a TTP > 50 s. The $\Delta T2^*_{max}$ has to be interpreted carefully since it is greatly influenced by O_2 extraction rate [13] and blood volume effects [11]. It is thought that due to lower flow rates, oxygen extraction is higher in PAD patients, therefore causing lower T2* signal gain. This is further accentuated by decreased blood pool within the region of interest (ROI) analyzed since PAD patients have decreased capillary density [14]. On the other hand, TTP is more specific and minimally affected by factors other than changes in perfusion [10,11].

The interscan and interobserver reproducibility of BOLD MRI was studied by Versluis et al. in 8 PAD patients and 10 normal volunteers using cuff occlusion [15]. Again, TTP was significantly prolonged in PAD patients compared to normal volunteers, but there was no difference in $\Delta T2^*_{max}$. Their results revealed that TTP was reasonably reproducible with an ICC of 0.80 and 0.69 for PAD patients and normal volunteers, respectively. The interobserver ICC for TTP was 0.78 and 0.59 for PAD patients and normal volunteers, respectively. The $\Delta T2^*_{max}$ had similar interscan reproducibility (ICC of 0.71 and 0.79 for PAD patients and volunteers) but better interobserver reproducibility (ICC of 0.99 for both groups). The study was limited by inclusion of large vessels in the analyzed ROI which can lead to inflow artifacts.

Susceptibility-Weighted MR Oximetry

Intravascular blood oxygen saturation can be quantified by MR oximetry using any one of three techniques sensitive to the volume fraction of deoxyhemoglobin: T2 [16], T2* [17] or magnetic susceptibility-weighted imaging (SWI) [18]. SWI oximetry is a calibration-free, T2*-sensitive method that uses both magnitude and phase information [18]. The magnetic susceptibility of blood is determined by the volume fraction of the paramagnetic deoxyhemoglobin in red blood cells and scales linearly with $(1 - HbO_2)$. Under normal conditions, tissue oxygen debt created by periods of ischemia due to arterial occlusion is followed by reactive hyperemia and increased oxygen uptake [19]. As such, repeated measurements of venous oxygen saturation following a period of hypoxia reflect the rate at which deoxygenated blood is replaced.

Langham et al. measured the change of oxygen saturation in the femoral/popliteal artery and vein during postocclusion reactive hyperemia in 10 young healthy (YH) volunteers, 12 PAD patients, and 8 age-matched healthy (AHC) volunteers [20]. To assess the contribution of the duration of hypoxia to the characteristics of reactive hyperemia, two occlusion periods of 3 and 5 min were used. Three parameters characterizing different temporal phases of reactivity were derived: washout time, defined as the time to lowest venous oxygen saturation; upslope, the slope from lowest saturation level to peak saturation level; and overshoot, peak oxygen saturation level achieved after washout (Fig. 7.5). PAD patients had longer washout time and lower upslope

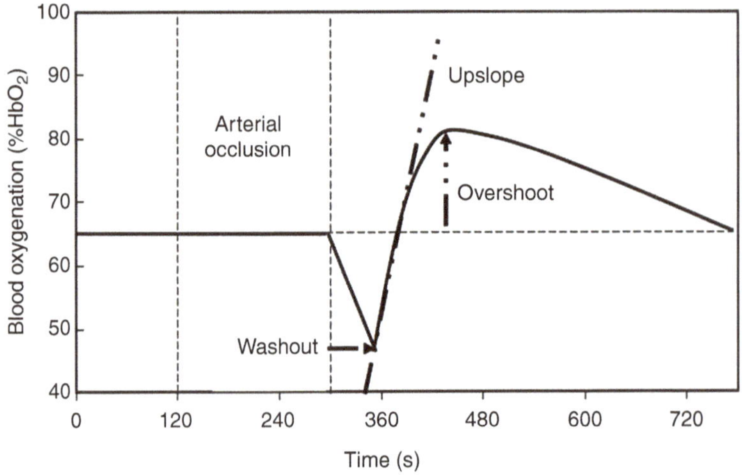

FIGURE 7.5 **Schematic of temporal changes in SvO_2 and parameters derived for quantifying reactive hyperemia.** *Dashed vertical lines* represent the beginning and end of cuff occlusion. *(Reproduced with permission [20].)*

compared to normal volunteers. Neither washout time nor upslope differed significantly. The reproducibility of SWI oximetry in PAD patients has not been rigorously studied.

MR Spectroscopic Measures of Tissue Energetics

^{31}Phosphorus (P) MR spectroscopy (MRS) allows in vivo measurements of the relative tissue concentrations of phosphocreatine (PCr), adenosinetriphosphate (ATP), and inorganic phosphate (P_i) in an imaging slab. PCr is the main energy reservoir and energy transport molecule of skeletal muscle. At the start of exercise, PCr is hydrolyzed via the creatine kinase pathway to synthesize ATP. The regeneration of PCr at the cessation of exercise occurs exclusively within the mitochondria and depends on the cell's oxidative phosphorylation capacity and oxygen supply [21]. Hence exercise is used for ^{31}P MRS testing. Multiple kinetic parameters can be characterized before, during, and after exercise. The PCr recovery time constant, a monoexponential fit of PCr levels versus time (beginning at the end of exercise), has been the most studied metric of mitochondrial function in PAD.

Several ^{31}P MRS studies have shown that the PCr recovery time constant is significantly prolonged in PAD patients compared to normal volunteers regardless of the exercise protocol used. Pipinos et al. tested 12 PAD patients and 14 normal volunteers using low workload isometric exercise [22]. They found that PCr and adenosinediphosphate (ADP) recovery time constants of PAD patients were significantly longer compared to normal volunteers. Using symptom-limited exercise, Isbell et al. showed that PCr recovery time constant clearly differentiates PAD patients from normal volunteers with area under the ROC curve of 0.925 ± 0.045 [23]. Additionally, the PCr recovery time constant was highly reproducible in both normal volunteers and PAD patients with an ICC of 0.95. There was no correlation with the screening ABI.

Combined Approaches

One group has put three MRI approaches together into a single MRI pulse sequence, combining measures of perfusion, intravenous oxygen saturation, and T2* (equivalent to BOLD) or PIVOT that was piloted in healthy controls during cuff occlusion and hyperemia [24]. PIVOT has a temporal resolution of 2 s and thus can measure the kinetics of perfusion, venous oxygenation, and T2*. In a recent study, 96 patients with PAD and 10 healthy controls were examined with PIVOT. Peak values for perfusion were all lower and TTP perfusion and T2* longer in PAD than controls. Increases in TTP for all three measures correlated inversely to the ABI. However, peak perfusion values did not correspond to the ABI, which is not surprising since the ABI measures bulk arterial flow and does not take collateral flow into account. The authors demonstrate that the most reliable measures were TTP perfusion and TTP T2*. What is not clear from this study is whether three techniques truly perform better than any one of these alone [25]. Venous blood oxygenation was only measurable in 77% of patients. The two TTP measures may be effectively measuring the same thing and their reproducibility was modest. Further studies are needed to sort out which of these is best applied to clinical trials.

Limitations

There are limitations to the use of MRI in some PAD patients. Patients with contraindications to MRI such as implanted cardioverter defibrillators, pacemakers, or those with claustrophobia are not candidates. In addition, patients with renal impairment (stage 4 or 5 chronic kidney disease, GFR < 30 mL/min/1.73 m2) and those with acute kidney injury cannot be studied with gadolinium-enhanced MRI due to the risk of nephrogenic systemic fibrosis [26]. ^{31}P spectroscopy is not available on all MRI scanners and thus is limited in its potential clinical applicability.

CONTRAST-ENHANCED ULTRASOUND

Contrast Ultrasound Imaging Technology

Agitated saline contrast has been used for several decades for the detection of right-to-left shunts and for the enhancement of Doppler signals for right-sided valves. The nitrogen and oxygen bubbles that are formed by hand agitation of saline or saline-blood mixtures are nonencapsulated, are too large, and are too short-lived to be used for opacifying the systemic blood pool or tissue perfusion [27]. Accordingly, the field of contrast echocardiography with more stable ultrasound contrast agents was developed with the overall goal of opacification the entire blood pool but has also been used to assess tissue perfusion [28,29]. The in vivo stability of microbubble (MB) contrast agents has been achieved by two approaches. Encapsulation of the MBs using lipid surfactant or albumin shells effectively reduces outward diffusion and deflation of MBs during their intravascular lifespan [28]. This encapsulation also reduces MB surface tension. Further improvement in MB stability has been afforded by using high-molecular weight gases such as perfluorocarbons [octafluoropropane (C_3F_8), decafluorobutane (C_4F_{10})] or sulfur hexafluoride (SF_6). Because these gases have low solubility (low Ostwald coefficient) and low diffusivity, they also prevent deflation in vivo which markedly increases their lifespan [30]. A partial list of MB agents approved for use in humans provided in Table 7.1.

For perfusion imaging, it is necessary to detect MB contrast agent within the microcirculation of the tissue. The most commonly used contrast imaging schemes rely on the detection of specific acoustic signatures produced by nonlinear oscillation MBs in the alternating pressure environment of the acoustic field [28,31]. Nonlinear oscillation occurs when MB vibration is eccentric with regards to extent and timing of the expansion and contraction regimes and is not linearly related to the applied US pressure. One of the most basic approaches is to simply filter received signals to those produced at twice the fundamental (transmission) frequency, often second harmonic imaging [32]. However, tissue can still produce backscatter at the second harmonic frequency. Accordingly, multipulse techniques have been used and described elsewhere which eliminate most tissue signal at either the fundamental or harmonic frequency range by comparing subtraction of pulses performed with acoustic phase-inversion or compounding pulses produced at different acoustic pressures [28,31]. These

TABLE 7.1 Commercially-Produced Microbubble Contrast Agents for Ultrasound

Shell composition	Gas	Size	Proprietary name
Lipid	C_3F_8	1–3 μm	Definity
	C_4F_{10}	2 μm	Sonazoid
	SF_6	2–3 μm	Sonovue/Lumason
	Air	2–3 μm	Levovist
Albumin	C_3F_8	2–4 μm	Optison
Polymer (PLGA)	PFC	2–3 μm	AI-700
Polymer/albumin	Air	2–3 μm	Cardiosphere

PFC, perfluorocarbon gas (not disclosed); *PLGA*, polylactide-*co*-glycolate.

approaches produce sufficient MB signal-to-noise relative to tissue to allow robust tissue-perfusion quantification.

Perfusion Imaging With Contrast-Enhanced Ultrasound

CEU perfusion imaging relies on the measurement of tissue blood flow using temporal data of contrast enhancement. The basis for CEU perfusion imaging is that MB contrast agents are pure intravascular tracers and have an identical rheologic behavior in the microcirculation as erythrocytes [33]. In the absence of any kinetic information, the degree of contrast enhancement in any tissue is directly proportional to that tissue's relative microvascular blood volume (the mass fraction that is attributable to actively perfused vasculature within the tissue of interest). Absolute blood volume which can be useful for assessing vascular responses to proangiogenic therapies can then be quantified in terms of mL/g of tissue by the knowledge of signal intensity for the blood pool as long as signal intensity is within the portion of the dynamic range where the relationship between MB concentration and intensity is predictable [28].

For the measurement of tissue blood flow, kinetic information is necessary. Two general approaches have been used. The first is to measure tissue transit rate kinetics after a bolus injection. This approach is advantageous in its simplicity. However, transit rate reflects not only blood flow but rather also the ratio of flow to microvascular volume so that analysis of blood volume becomes necessary [34]. Moreover, transit rate is also influence by the input function (the contrast entry profile from the main arterial inflow) which is not easily measured by CEU and is influenced by injection speed and cardiac output. Another approach is to use contrast destruction-replenishment kinetics whereby contrast agents are infused continuously and the rate and extent of contrast reappearance in the tissue of interest are used to calculate myocardial microvascular blood flux rate and microvascular blood volume in a matter of seconds [29]. The product of these two parameters is equivalent to microvascular blood flow. The only major limitation of this approach is the lower signal intensity achieved compared to bolus techniques which can present a problem when imaging tissues with extremely low blood flow at rest (<0.1 mL/min/g).

CEU Perfusion Imaging in PAD

The application of CEU for evaluation of PAD is an attractive approach because of practical considerations of cost, speed, and the preexisting presence of ultrasound in vascular laboratories. Moreover, CEU is able to assess flow quantitatively rather than measuring spatial heterogeneity of flow which is a particular concern for assessing PAD and less so for coronary artery disease. Accordingly, both bolus transit rate analysis and destruction-replenishment kinetics have been used to measure perfusion at rest or during stress to assess limb ischemia in PAD [35,36].

Early studies using transit rate analysis were performed in subjects with intermittent claudication (ie, Rutherford class I-III) as a manifestation of their PAD [35,37]. Despite the fact that these patients did not have any resting symptoms, CEU performed at rest demonstrated significant differences between patients and control subjects in the temporal domain parameter of time-to-peak after bolus injection [35]. There was also a clear separation between cohorts for time-to-peak during contractile exercise, although the approximate amount of "flow reserve" by this parameter did not appear to be different between groups. The parameter of time-to-peak also did not correlate with ABI which indicates dissociation between pressure drop in the conduit artery and tissue perfusion that has been consistent among studies. Another study performed in the same type of patient population used a variant of transit rate analysis by comparing contrast wash-in curves during the immediate hyperemic phase after releasing a cuff that occluded arterial inflow for 1 min [37]. This study also showed significant differences between PAD patients and controls with respect to time-to-peak contrast as well as peak contrast enhancement.

Bolus transit rate analysis has also been investigated with regards to the ability to quantify the severity of perfusion defects and response to therapy. In a study of patients with claudication or critical limb ischemia (Fontaine Class IIa to IV), time-to-peak contrast tended to increase with the symptomatic severity of disease (Fig. 7.6) [38]. Moreover, in those with severe disease the time-to-peak tended to be longest in those with poor collateralization. Again, there was no relationship between ABI and the CEU data. The time-to-peak function after contrast bolus has also been used to demonstrate improvement in microvascular flow after either surgical or percutaneous revascularization [39]. In this study,

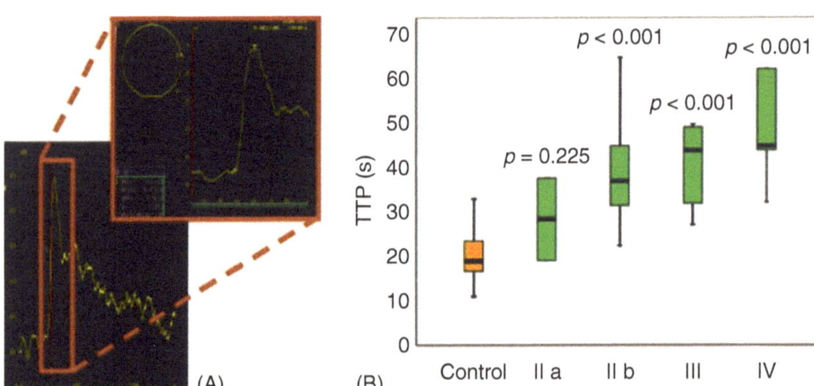

FIGURE 7.6 CEU time-intensity analysis from calf muscle after intravenous bolus injection of contrast agent in patients with PAD. (A) Illustration of an entire time-intensity plot expanded time scale of the appearance phase for contrast after intravenous injection. (B) Box-whisker plot of the TTP of contrast appearance for control subjects and patients with different Fontaine grades for severity of PAD (p-values are relative to control subjects). *(Reproduced with permission from Ref. [38].)*

however, there was no demonstrated advantage of CEU to ABI with regards to detecting a change from pre- to postrevascularization.

The CEU destruction-replenishment approach to measuring tissue perfusion has been the most popular approach for ischemic heart disease due to the ability to quantify tissue perfusion. Its application for evaluating PAD was based on results from a canine study of graded femoral artery stenosis [40]. In this study, during contractile exercise there was a stepwise reduction in microvascular blood flow with increasing degrees of stenosis. Moreover, resting hypoperfusion could also be detected in the presence of moderate to severe stenosis (transstenotic pressure gradients of 25–35 mmHg). These results led to a clinical study where CEU perfusion imaging with destruction-replenishment kinetics was performed in control subjects and PAD patients with intermittent claudication [36]. Compared with control subjects, those with PAD had lower exercise limb perfusion on CEU and lower limb perfusion reserve. There were two findings that suggested a particularly strong role of CEU. The first was that perfusion during exercise was still markedly abnormal in those with PAD and claudication but who had an ABI > 0.9. Second, PAD patients with diabetes mellitus who are recognized to have microvascular abnormalities that compound large inflow vessel disease were characterized by particularly poor perfusion. Perhaps the most important data were that CEU perfusion during exercise or flow reserve were better predictors of the severity of symptoms (assessed by time to symptoms on upright treadmill exercise test) than were traditional measures such as ABI, exercise ABI, and pulse-volume recordings.

CEU Assessment of Cell Therapy for PAD

Currently, CEU perfusion imaging has been used as a biologic readout for cell-based proangiogenic therapy only in preclinical models of disease. The foundation for these studies lies in experimental data that have shown that CEU allows precise measurement of changes in tissue perfusion in response to established (eg, revascularization) or experimental (eg, gene therapy) therapies that are aimed at improving tissue perfusion [39,41–43]. With regards to proangiogenic gene therapy, CEU using the destruction-replenishment technique has been particularly useful in decoding the vascular responses. The ability of CEU destruction-replenishment algorithms to parametrically assess microvascular blood volume and microvascular flux rate allows one to assess the relative contributions of adding functional microvascular units and changing total network vascular conductance [43,44]. Moreover, CEU data can be modeled to differentially assess increases in vascular blood volume at the capillary level (arteriogenesis) and remodeling at the on-capillary microcirculation which generally reflects arteriogenesis or arteriolar remodeling [44].

The ability to temporally assess the effects of cell therapy using CEU has been demonstrated in a murine model of chronic hindlimb ischemia (Fig. 7.7) [45]. In these studies, CEU was performed after administration of a type of

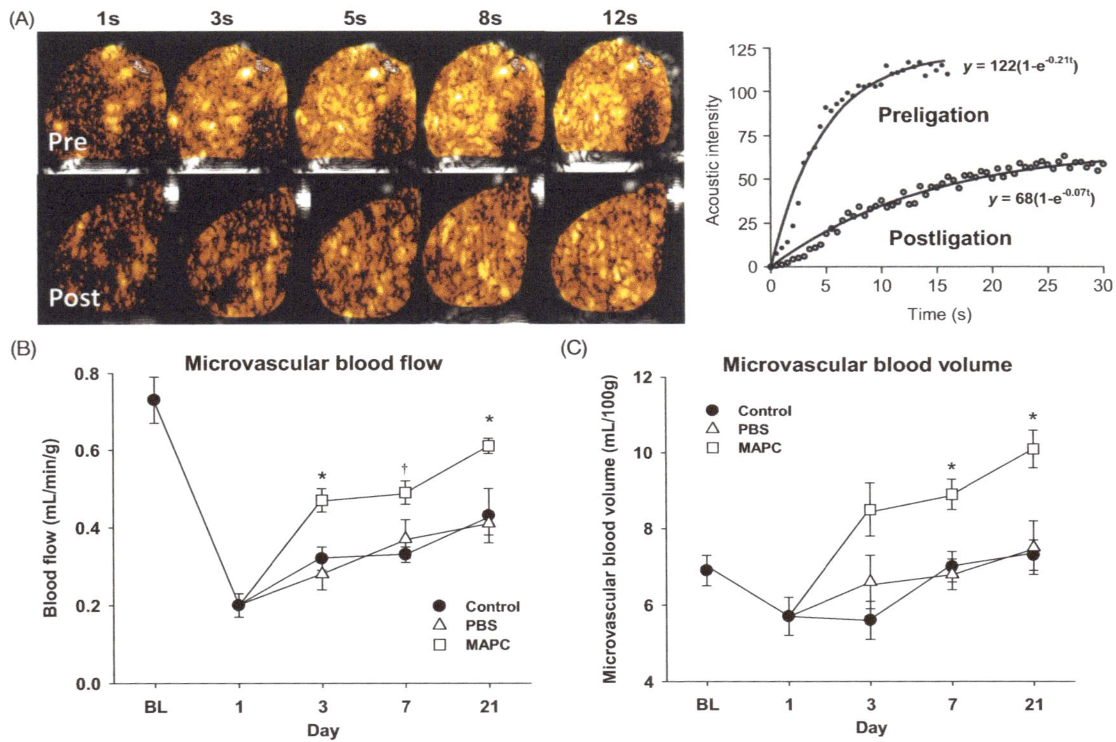

FIGURE 7.7 **CEU evaluation of perfusion in response to cell therapy.** (A) Examples of time-intensity data and corresponding background-subtracted color-coded images from murine proximal hindlimb skeletal muscle illustrating ischemia produced by arterial ligation. (B and C) Quantitative CEU data from the proximal hindlimb demonstrating augmentation in flow recovery and expansion of the intramuscular microvascular blood volume in animals receiving intramuscular administration of multipotential adult progenitor cells (MAPC) at day 1 after arterial ligation. PBS, sham-treated control limbs treated with PBS intramuscularly. $^{*}p < 0.05$ versus both control groups; $^{\dagger}p < 0.05$ versus control nontreated. *(Reproduced with permission from Ref. [45].)*

adult mesenchymal stem cell (multipotential adult progenitor cells) administered by intramuscular route. In this study, microvascular blood flow (in mL/min/g) and measurements made by CEU demonstrated significant increases in perfusion at days 3, 7, and 21 after cell therapy. Microvascular blood volume measured by CEU after cell therapy not only increased but exceeded baseline levels which correlated on postmortem histology with remodeling of the arteriolar network.

Limitations

Although CEU is thought to be not only an accurate but also practical method for assessing changes in perfusion with cell therapy, robust clinical data are lacking. Only recently has there been a single case report using CEU in a patient with critical limb ischemia undergoing limb injection of cord blood-derived mononuclear cells [46]. Also, although ultrasound appears to be clinically convenient because of the existing presence of ultrasound imaging systems in most vascular laboratories, specialized software for contrast-specific imaging is generally required and perfusion imaging is considered an off-label use for MB agents.

RADIONUCLIDE IMAGING

Radionuclide Imaging Technology

Over the last several decades, advancements in RNI techniques including radioisotope tracer design and sensitivity and resolution of detectors (eg, iterative reconstruction, cadmium-zinc-telluride detectors, etc.) have made these modalities an integral part of the diagnostic workup and management of patients with coronary artery disease (CAD) [47,48]. These techniques have not had much role in the evaluation of subjects with PAD, although there is renewed interest in this potential application. Reasons for this discrepancy in use for two different manifestations of obstructive atherosclerotic disease (CAD vs PAD) include the practical considerations of cost, time, and exposure to relatively high doses of radionuclide tracers. However, a more important consideration is the difference between these two conditions in the regional variation of perfusion. For CAD, the easiest and most commonly employed algorithm is to evaluate relative regional myocardial tracer uptake on PET or single-photon emission computed tomography (SPECT). Quantification of RNI in most high-throughput clinical laboratories simply relies on the comparing relative regional uptake patterns to normative databases on the basis of gender and body morphometry. Regional heterogeneity in CAD is based on the premise that the most common manifestation of CAD involves nonuniform stenosis in the three major coronary arterial distributions. Even in the setting where the degree of ischemia is relative uniform, there are other indicators that can be used to recognize the presence of three-vessel CAD such as transient ischemic dilation or evidence for stunning on gated SPECT [49]. In PAD, however, the high likelihood of disease in large single inflow conduit arteries that supply very large relative distributions diffuse or disease in every major branching conduit vessel makes the approach of evaluating relative tracer insensitive for detection of PAD or for assessing the effects of revascularization. However, the advent of perfusion imaging quantification techniques and relative uptake values for not only PET but also SPECT increases the feasibility for using RNI for not only research protocols but also for clinical imaging [50].

Assessment of Flow and Perfusion

Most of the early RNI experience in measuring total limb and regional blood flow had been assessed on the basis of the clearance rate of intramuscular injections of ^{99m}Tc-pertechnetate and ^{133}Xe [51,52]. However, this approach lacked accuracy since clearance of these tracers is influenced by much more than simply microvascular perfusion (eg, injection volume/site, lymphatic clearance, etc.). First-pass transit rate kinetics similar to that performed with MRI and CEU have also been examined using tracers such as radiolabeled albumin [53]. However, these techniques require arterial injection due to lack of ability to deconvolve the input function and, as discussed previously, provide information primarily on flow per microvascular volume rather than flow itself.

More conventional MPI techniques have been applied to limb imaging with SPECT agents such as ^{201}Tl and the host of ^{99m}Tc-labeled agents that have been developed for cardiac imaging [50,54]. In particular, agents with high first-pass extraction are advantageous for use in limb skeletal muscle imaging due to the low blood flow at rest in skeletal muscle. Moreover, stress–rest imaging algorithms can be performed similar to that used for CAD. Although regional differences in general muscle locations can be detected with SPECT MPI and tend to be more pronounced in PAD, most studies with SPECT tracers involve either evaluation relative to a normal limb or in comparison to total body uptake in those with rather severe disease, all of which makes quantitative measures of perfusion abnormalities with SPECT rather coarse and sometimes inaccurate if there is either mild disease or diffuse atherosclerotic disease involving many sites in the body [55,56]. However there are data that also suggest that quantitative rest-exercise stress SPECT can detect subclinical PAD in diabetic patients who do not necessarily exhibit abnormalities in ankle–brachial index [57].

Because of the need to quantify perfusion in bilateral PAD, PET is a somewhat more attractive alternative due to the established algorithms for perfusion quantification, particularly with the freely diffusible short-half-life tracer $^{15}O\text{-}H_2O$. Using this tracer, studies have demonstrated the efficacy of PET in detecting the presence of PAD [58,59]. Studies comparing PET to microsphere-derived blood flow in animal models and to thermodilution in humans (11) have demonstrated that flow reserve can be accurately measured which is important for the evaluation of patients with IC rather than CLI [60,61]. However the cost, availability, and short half-life of most of the PET tracers that have been used for perfusion imaging may very well limit their widespread adoption as a clinical tool.

It is also important to realize that PET imaging has the capability of assessing metabolic processes that can reflect the underlying tissue responses or consequences of ischemia. PET imaging methods have been developed to detect muscle tissue hypoxia (eg, ^{18}F-MISO) and altered metabolism (glucose versus fatty acid; oxidative pathways with ^{11}C-acetate) [62]. The potential of these applications in PAD assessment have not yet been fully explored.

Radionuclide Imaging of Angiogenesis and Cell Therapy

Imaging of angiogenesis with RNI in animal models of disease, and even in humans in preliminary trials, has been mostly relegated to molecular imaging of vascular remodeling (eg, VEGF receptors, ischemia-related integrins such as $\alpha_v\beta_3$, or components of the inflammatory response) which is out of the scope of this chapter [50]. The RNI techniques described previously have been used not infrequently to quantitatively assess changes in perfusion defect size in angiogenesis trials in the myocardium. However, they have only rarely been used in preclinical models of therapeutic angiogenesis and mostly as an adjunct to document recovery of limb blood flow in studies primarily designed to evaluate the performance of molecular targeted agents [63]. However, recent studies using SPECT 201-Tl perfusion imaging (normalized to a contralateral limb) in animal models of endogenous angiogenesis have indicated that this approach correlates to histologic evidence of angiogenesis and CT-angiography evidence for arteriogenesis (Fig. 7.8) [64].

With regards to cell therapy for therapeutic angiogenesis in PAD, much of the application of RNI has been to temporally assess the biodistribution and survival of stem cells using either radionuclide tracer loading of stem cells or genetic modification of stem cells to enable their intracellular retention of a molecular imaging tracer that is administered by intravenous route [65]. The use of RNI perfusion imaging to serially quantify the biologic effects of cell therapy in PAD remains an unmet potential.

Limitations

As with the other imaging modalities, the primary limitation of RNI is the limited experience to date using the technique to assess microvascular response to proangiogenic therapies. Moreover, because of the diffuse nature of atherosclerotic disease, sophisticated quantitative algorithms are more apt to provide valuable information rather than relative uptake of tracer between different anatomic beds.

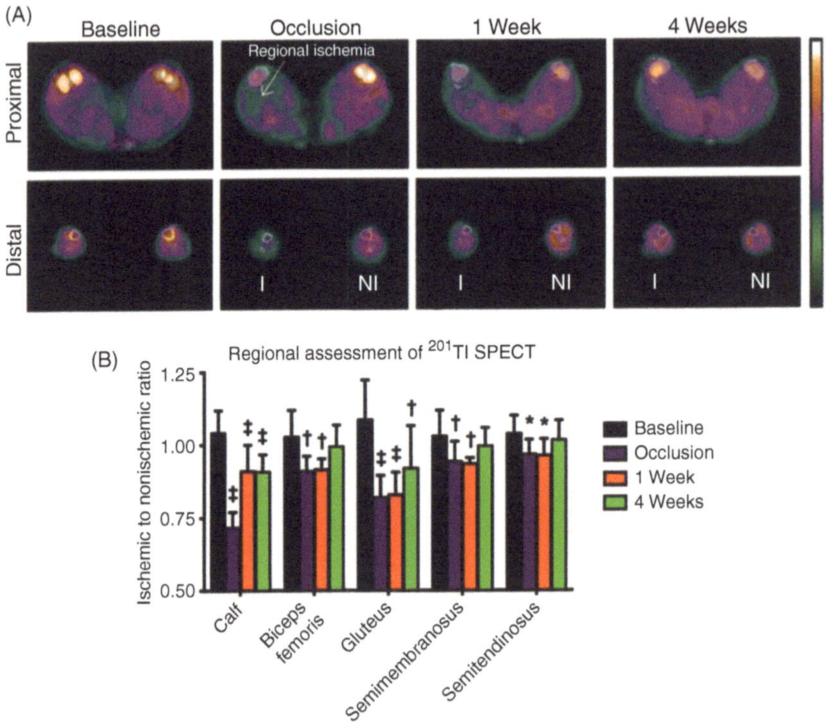

FIGURE 7.8 **Quantification of endogenous angiogenesis with 201-Thallium SPECT/CT imaging in a porcine model of femoral ligation.** (A) SPECT images demonstrating a perfusion defect in the proximal (top row) and distal (bottom row) hindlimb which decrease in severity over time (arrow depicts muscle group of interest). (B) Quantitative RNI activity of different muscle groups relative to the contralateral limb over time demonstrating flow recovery over 4 weeks. $^{*}p < 0.05$; $^{\dagger}p < 0.01$; $^{\ddagger}p < 0.0001$ versus baseline. *(Reproduced with permission from Ref. [64].)*

CONCLUSIONS

MRI, CEU, and radionuclide techniques offer promise in the assessment of angiogenic and stem cell therapy. None have been studied to date in large-scale clinical trials. In addition, no head-to-head comparison of any these techniques is available to demonstrate which might be best used in trials of regenerative therapy. Each may measure different physiological parameters and may not necessarily correlate with each other. For example, PCr recovery kinetics and first-pass perfusion CE-MRI each correlate with functional performance (treadmill time or 6-min walk, respectively) but do not correlate with each other [66]. Some techniques may work best in concert with others. Regardless, the future of imaging of angiogenic therapy and stem cell therapy in PAD appears bright.

REFERENCES

[1] Wilke N, Simm C, Zhang J, et al. Contrast-enhanced first pass myocardial perfusion imaging: correlation between myocardial blood flow in dogs at rest and during hyperemia. Magn Reson Med 1993;29:485–97.

[2] Epstein FH, London JF, Peters DC, et al. Multislice first-pass cardiac perfusion MRI: validation in a model of myocardial infarction. Magn Reson Med 2002;47:482–91.

[3] Thompson RB, Aviles RJ, Faranesh AZ, et al. Measurement of skeletal muscle perfusion during postischemic reactive hyperemia using contrast-enhanced MRI with a step-input function. Magn Reson Med 2005;54(2):289–98.

[4] Isbell DC, Epstein FH, Zhong X, et al. Calf muscle perfusion at peak exercise in peripheral arterial disease: measurement by first pass contrast-enhanced magnetic resonance imaging. J Magn Reson Imaging 2007;25:1013–20.

[5] Jiji RS, Pollak AW, Epstein FH, et al. Reproducibility of rest and exercise stress contrast-enhanced calf perfusion magnetic resonance imaging in peripheral arterial disease. J Cardiovasc Magn Reson 2013;15:14.

[6] Raynaud JS, Duteil S, Vaughan JT, et al. Determination of skeletal muscle perfusion using arterial spin labeling NMRI: validation by comparison with venous occlusion plethysmography. Magn Reson Med 2001 August;46:305–11.

[7] Wu WC, Mohler E III, Ratcliffe SJ, Wehrli FW, Detre JA, Floyd TF. Skeletal muscle microvascular flow in progressive peripheral artery disease: assessment with continuous arterial spin-labeling perfusion magnetic resonance imaging. J Am Coll Cardiol 2009;53(25):2372–7.

[8] Pollak AW, Meyer CH, Epstein FH, et al. Arterial spin labeling MRI reproducibly measures peak-exercise calf muscle perfusion in healthy volunteers and patients with peripheral arterial disease. JACC Cardiovasc Imaging 2012;5(12):1224–30.

[9] Jacobi B, Bongartz G, Partovi S, et al. Skeletal muscle BOLD MRI: from underlying physiological concepts to its usefulness in clinical conditions. J Magn Reson Imaging 2012;35(6):1253–65.

[10] Lebon V, Carlier PG, Brillault-Salvat C, Leroy-Willig A. Simultaneous measurement of perfusion and oxygenation changes using a multiple gradient-echo sequence: application to human muscle study. Magn Reson Imaging 1998;16(7):721–9.

[11] Duteil S, Wary C, Raynaud JS, et al. Influence of vascular filling and perfusion on BOLD contrast during reactive hyperemia in human skeletal muscle. Magn Reson Med 2006;55:450–4.

[12] Ledermann H, Schulte AC, Heidecker HG, et al. Blood oxygenation level-dependent magnetic resonance imaging of the skeletal muscle in patients with peripheral arterial occlusive disease. Circulation 2006;113(25):2929–35.

[13] Logothetis NK, Wandell BA. Interpreting the BOLD Signal. Annu Rev Physiol 2004;66(1):735–69.

[14] Robbins JL, Jones WS, Duscha BD, et al. Relationship between leg muscle capillary density and peak hyperemic blood flow with endurance capacity in peripheral artery disease. J Appl Physiol 2011;111(1):81–6.

[15] Versluis B, Backes WH, van Eupen MGA, et al. Magnetic resonance imaging in peripheral arterial disease: reproducibility of the assessment of morphological and functional vascular status. Invest Radiol 2011;46(1).

[16] Wright GA, Hu BS, Macovski A. Estimating oxygen saturation of blood in vivo with MR imaging at 1.5 T. J Magn Reson Imaging 1991;1(3):275–83.

[17] Chien D, Levin DL, Anderson CM. MR gradient echo imaging of intravascular blood oxygenation: T2* determination in the presence of flow. Magn Reson Med 1994;32(4):540–5.

[18] Haacke EM, Lai S, Reichenbach JR, et al. In vivo measurement of blood oxygen saturation using magnetic resonance imaging: a direct validation of the blood oxygen level-dependent concept in functional brain imaging. Hum Brain Mapp 1997;5(5):341–6.
[19] Abramson DI, Tuck S, Bell Y, Mitchell RE, Zayas AM. Effect of short periods of arterial occlusion on blood flow and oxygen uptake. J Appl Physiol 1961;16(5):851–7.
[20] Langham MC, Floyd T, Mohler ER, Magland JF, Wehrli FW. Evaluation of cuff-induced ischemia in the lower extremity by magnetic resonance oximetry. J Am Coll Cardiol 2010;55(6):598–606.
[21] Bessman SP, Geiger PJ. Transport of energy in muscle: the phosphorylcreatine shuttle. Science 1981;211:448–52.
[22] Pipinos II, Shepard AD, Anagnostopoulos PV, Katsamouris A, Boska MD. Phophorus 31 nuclear magnetic resonance spectroscopy suggests a mitochondrial defect in claudicating skeletal muscle. J Vasc Surg 2000;31:944–52.
[23] Isbell DC, Berr SS, Toledano AY, et al. Delayed calf muscle phosphocreatine recovery after exercise identifies peripheral arterial disease. J Am Coll Cardiol 2006;47(11):2289–97.
[24] Englund EK, Langham MC, Li C, et al. Combined measurement of perfusion, venous oxygen saturation, and skeletal muscle T(2)* during reactive hyperemia in the leg. J Cardiovasc Magn Reson 2013;15(1):70.
[25] Kramer CM. Novel magnetic resonance imaging end points for physiologic studies in peripheral arterial disease: elegance versus practicality. Circ Cardiovasc Imaging 2015;8(4).
[26] Kaewlai R, Abujudeh H. Nephrogenic systemic fibrosis. AJR 2012;199(1):W17–23.
[27] Jeon DS, Luo H, Iwami T, Miyamoto T, Brasch AV, Mirocha J, et al. The usefulness of a 10% air-10% blood-80% saline mixture for contrast echocardiography: Doppler measurement of pulmonary artery systolic pressure. J Am Coll Cardiol. 2002;39:124–9.
[28] Lindner JR, Wei K. Contrast echocardiography. Curr Probl Cardiol 2002;27:454–519.
[29] Wei K, Jayaweera AR, Firoozan S, Linka A, Skyba DM, Kaul S. Quantification of myocardial blood flow with ultrasound-induced destruction of microbubbles administered as a constant venous infusion. Circulation 1998;97:473–83.
[30] Kabalnov A, Klein D, Pelura T, Schutt E, Weers J. Dissolution of multicomponent microbubbles in the bloodstream: 1. Theory. Ultrasound Med Biol 1998;24:739–49.
[31] Eckersley RJ, Chin CT, Burns PN. Optimising phase and amplitude modulation schemes for imaging microbubble contrast agents at low acoustic power. Ultrasound Med Biol 2005;31:213–9.
[32] Burns PN. Harmonic imaging with ultrasound contrast agents. Clin Radiol 1996;51 (Suppl 1):50–5.
[33] Lindner JR, Song J, Jayaweera AR, Sklenar J, Kaul S. Microvascular rheology of definity microbubbles after intra-arterial and intravenous administration. J Am Soc Echocardiogr 2002;15:396–403.
[34] Lindner JR, Skyba DM, Goodman NC, Jayaweera AR, Kaul S. Changes in myocardial blood volume with graded coronary stenosis. Am J Physiol 1997;272:H567–75.
[35] Duerschmied D, Olson L, Olschewski M, Rossknecht A, Freund G, Bode C, et al. Contrast ultrasound perfusion imaging of lower extremities in peripheral arterial disease: a novel diagnostic method. Eur Heart J 2006;27:310–5.
[36] Lindner JR, Womack L, Barrett EJ, Weltman J, Price W, Harthun NL, et al. Limb stress-rest perfusion imaging with contrast ultrasound for the assessment of peripheral arterial disease severity. JACC Cardiovasc Imaging 2008;1:343–50.
[37] Amarteifio E, Weber MA, Wormsbecher S, Demirel S, Krakowski-Roosen H, Jores A, et al. Dynamic contrast-enhanced ultrasound for assessment of skeletal muscle microcirculation in peripheral arterial disease. Invest Radiol 2011;46:504–8.

[38] Duerschmied D, Zhou Q, Rink E, Harder D, Freund G, Olschewski M, et al. Simplified contrast ultrasound accurately reveals muscle perfusion deficits and reflects collateralization in pad. Atherosclerosis 2009;202:505–12.

[39] Duerschmied D, Maletzki P, Freund G, Olschewski M, Bode C, Hehrlein C. Success of arterial revascularization determined by contrast ultrasound muscle perfusion imaging. J Vasc Surg 2010;52:1531–6.

[40] Bragadeesh T, Sari I, Pascotto M, Micari A, Kaul S, Lindner JR. Detection of peripheral vascular stenosis by assessing skeletal muscle flow reserve. J Am Coll Cardiol 2005;45:780–5.

[41] Kuliszewski MA, Kobulnik J, Lindner JR, Stewart DJ, Leong-Poi H. Vascular gene transfer of sdf-1 promotes endothelial progenitor cell engraftment and enhances angiogenesis in ischemic muscle. Mol Ther 2011;19:895–902.

[42] Leong-Poi H, Kuliszewski MA, Lekas M, Sibbald M, Teichert-Kuliszewska K, Klibanov AL, et al. Therapeutic arteriogenesis by ultrasound-mediated vegf165 plasmid gene delivery to chronically ischemic skeletal muscle. Circ Res 2007;101:295–303.

[43] Leong-Poi H, Christiansen J, Heppner P, Lewis CW, Klibanov AL, Kaul S, et al. Assessment of endogenous and therapeutic arteriogenesis by contrast ultrasound molecular imaging of integrin expression. Circulation 2005;111:3248–54.

[44] Pascotto M, Leong-Poi H, Kaufmann B, Allrogen A, Charalampidis D, Kerut EK, et al. Assessment of ischemia-induced microvascular remodeling using contrast-enhanced ultrasound vascular anatomic mapping. J Am Soc Echocardiogr 2007;20:1100–8.

[45] Ryu JC, Davidson BP, Xie A, Qi Y, Zha D, Belcik JT, et al. Molecular imaging of the paracrine proangiogenic effects of progenitor cell therapy in limb ischemia. Circulation 2013;127:710–9.

[46] Perotti C, Arici V, Cervio M, Del Fante C, Calliada F, Gnecchi M, et al. Allogeneic lethally irradiated cord blood mononuclear cells in no-option critical limb ischemia: a "box of rain". Stem Cells Dev 2013;22:2806–12.

[47] Garcia EV. Physical attributes, limitations, and future potential for pet and spect. J Nucl Cardiol 2012;19(Suppl 1):S19–29.

[48] Maddahi J. Properties of an ideal pet perfusion tracer: new pet tracer cases and data. J Nucl Cardiol 2012;19(Suppl 1):S30–7.

[49] Hida S, Chikamori T, Tanaka H, Igarashi Y, Shiba C, Hatano T, et al. Postischemic myocardial stunning is superior to transient ischemic dilation for detecting multivessel coronary artery disease. Circ J 2012;76:430–8.

[50] Stacy MR, Zhou W, Sinusas AJ. Radiotracer imaging of peripheral vascular disease. J Nucl Med 2013;54:2104–10.

[51] Lassen NA, Lindbjerg J, Munck O. Measurement of blood-flow through skeletal muscle by intramuscular injection of xenon-133. Lancet 1964;1:686–9.

[52] Cutajar CL, Brown NJ, Marston A. Muscle blood-flow studies by the technetium (99mtc) clearance technique in normal subjects and in patients with intermittent claudication. Br J Surg 1971;58:532–7.

[53] Rhodes BA, Greyson ND, Siegel ME, Giargiana FA Jr, White RI Jr, Williams GM, et al. The distribution of radioactive microspheres after intra-arterial injection in the legs of patients with peripheral vascular disease. AJR 1973;118:820–6.

[54] Wolfram RM, Budinsky AC, Sinzinger H. Assessment of peripheral arterial vascular disease with radionuclide techniques. Semin Nucl Med 2001;31:129–42.

[55] Earnshaw JJ, Hardy JG, Hopkinson BR, Makin GS. Non-invasive investigation of lower limb revascularisation using resting thallium peripheral perfusion imaging. Eur J Nucl Med 1986;12:443–6.

[56] Hamanaka D, Odori T, Maeda H, Ishii Y, Hayakawa K, Torizuka K. A quantitative assessment of scintigraphy of the legs using 201tl. Eur J Nucl Med 1984;9:12–6.

[57] Duet M, Virally M, Bailliart O, Kevorkian JP, Kedra AW, Benelhadj S, et al. Whole-body (201)tl scintigraphy can detect exercise lower limb perfusion abnormalities in asymptomatic diabetic patients with normal doppler pressure indices. Nucl Med Commun 2001;22:949–54.
[58] Scremin OU, Figoni SF, Norman K, Scremin AM, Kunkel CF, Opava-Rutter D, et al. Preamputation evaluation of lower-limb skeletal muscle perfusion with h(2) (15)o positron emission tomography. Am J Phys Med Rehabil 2010;89:473–86.
[59] Depairon M, Zicot M. The quantitation of blood flow/metabolism coupling at rest and after exercise in peripheral arterial insufficiency, using pet and 15-0 labeled tracers. Angiology 1996;47:991–9.
[60] Schmidt MA, Chakrabarti A, Shamim-Uzzaman Q, Kaciroti N, Koeppe RA, Rajagopalan S. Calf flow reserve with h(2)(15)o pet as a quantifiable index of lower extremity flow. J Nucl Med 2003;44:915–9.
[61] Penuelas I, Aranguren XL, Abizanda G, Marti-Climent JM, Uriz M, Ecay M, et al. (13)*n*-ammonia pet as a measurement of hindlimb perfusion in a mouse model of peripheral artery occlusive disease. J Nucl Med 2007;48:1216–23.
[62] Peterson LR, Gropler RJ. Radionuclide imaging of myocardial metabolism. Circ Cardiovasc Imaging 2010;3:211–22.
[63] Orbay H, Zhang Y, Hong H, Hacker TA, Valdovinos HF, Zagzebski JA, et al. Positron emission tomography imaging of angiogenesis in a murine hindlimb ischemia model with 64cu-labeled trc105. Mol Pharm 2013;10:2749–56.
[64] Stacy MR, Yu da Y, Maxfield MW, Jaba IM, Jozwik BP, Zhuang ZW, et al. Multimodality imaging approach for serial assessment of regional changes in lower extremity arteriogenesis and tissue perfusion in a porcine model of peripheral arterial disease. Circ Cardiovasc Imaging 2014;7:92–9.
[65] Chen IY, Wu JC. Molecular imaging: the key to advancing cardiac stem cell therapy. Trends Cardiovasc Med 2013;23:201–10.
[66] Anderson JA, Epstein FH, Meyer CH, et al. Multifactorial determinants of functional capacity in peripheral arterial disease: uncoupling of calf muscle perfusion and metabolism. J Am Coll Cardiol 2009;54:628–34.

Chapter 8

Endpoint Assessment for Cell Therapy in Patients with Intermittent Claudication and Critical Limb Ischemia

W.S. Jones, MD, D. Kopin, MD
Department of Medicine, Duke University Medical Center, Durham, NC, United States

INTRODUCTION

Peripheral artery disease (PAD) affects over eight million Americans and is associated with significant morbidity and mortality as it is a marker of subclinical heart disease and systemic atherosclerosis [1]. Patients with PAD are at increased risk for myocardial infarction, stroke, and death [1–3]. PAD can be silent, however when symptomatic it is associated with a significant reduction in quality of life (QOL) and, in its most sobering form, limb amputation [1,2]. Given its substantial health burden, PAD has become the focus of many therapeutic developments including drugs, surgical revascularization, endovascular devices, and emerging gene and cellular therapies discussed in this book.

With the vast number of emerging treatments, it is clear that there is a strong need for high-quality clinical trials to help guide regulatory approval and practice guidelines aimed at providing clinicians with the tools to understand how to measure treatment outcomes and ultimately improve patient outcomes. However, unlike coronary artery disease, many clinical trials in patients with PAD variably collect and report baseline characteristics, disease severity, and treatment outcomes [4]. This presents a difficult issue for clinicians when comparing data between trials, especially since there are few direct comparative effectiveness studies available in the PAD literature. Many academic research organizations, professional societies, regulatory agencies, and pharmaceutical agencies have proposed standardized definitions for PAD populations, however, their broad application has been limited [5–7]. This chapter will discuss the most widely used definitions of the clinical symptoms, outcomes, and endpoints for patients with PAD and recommend standardization of them moving forward in order to improve consistency and validity between studies.

Regenerative Medicine for Peripheral Artery Disease. http://dx.doi.org/10.1016/B978-0-12-801344-1.00008-5

Very broadly, PAD results in limb ischemia and can manifest as either intermittent claudication (IC) or critical limb ischemia (CLI). Classically, IC is defined as exertional, ischemic leg pain that is relieved with rest. However, it is a heterogeneous disease and can also present with atypical leg symptoms including cramping; numbness; soreness; skin, hair, and nail changes; and coldness. Conversely, the hallmarks of CLI include ischemic rest pain, tissue ulceration, and gangrene.

It is crucial to define the most meaningful endpoints with regard to treatment of CLI and IC since many potential endpoints and much controversy regarding their importance exist. In general, meaningful endpoints for patients with PAD can be divided into cardiovascular endpoints (cardiovascular mortality, myocardial infarction, stroke), limb-specific endpoints (functional capacity, QOL, amputation, acute limb ischemia, wound healing, analog pain scale, and disease progression), and combination endpoints (amputation-free survival). It is also important to determine how these will be measured as this can drastically affect the way in which data is interpreted and ultimately the outcome and clinical impact of studies. This is especially important because despite the prevalence of PAD, recruiting subjects for randomized trials has been paradoxically slow and a common practice in clinical trials of PAD patients is to use historical controls as a comparator to eliminate issues with slow enrollment [8,9]. Another issue that has complicated clinical trials in the PAD field is the use of objective performance controls for single-arm comparisons for device evaluation, a practice that the US Food and Drug Administration has accepted. The use of historical controls and objective performance measures in clinical trials is not unique to the field of PAD, however, given the lack of standardized definitions and clinical endpoints that will be described in this chapter; their use in PAD trials is particularly problematic and makes it difficult to interpret results.

ENDPOINTS USED

It is difficult to define which endpoints are most useful with respect to IC and CLI. Generally studies investigating treatments for CLI and IC use some combination of the following endpoints:

- Cardiovascular events (including MI, stroke, and cardiovascular mortality)
- Functional capacity
- QOL
- Major and minor amputation
- Acute limb ischemia
- Wound healing
- Analog pain scale
- Disease progression as measured by a change in symptoms according to the Rutherford or Fontaine score (see Table 8.1)
- Amputation-free survival

TABLE 8.1 Clinical Classification for Patients With LE PAD

Fontaine classification		Proposed PARC universal data elements			Rutherford classification
Stage	Symptoms		Grade	Category	Symptoms
I	Asymptomatic	Asymptomatic	0	0	Asymptomatic
II	Intermittent claudication/ other exertional limb symptoms	Mild claudication/ limb symptoms (no limitation in walking)	1	1	Mild claudication
IIa		Moderate claudication/limb symptoms (able to walk without stopping ≥2 blocks or 200 m or 4 min)	1	2	Moderate claudication
IIb		Severe claudication/ limb symptoms (only able to walk without stopping <2 blocks or 200 m or 4 min)	1	3	Severe claudication
III	Ischemic rest pain	Ischemic rest pain (pain in the distal limb at rest felt to be due limited arterial perfusion)	2	4	Ischemic Rest Pain
IV	Ulceration or gangrene	Ischemic ulcers on distal leg	3	5	Ischemic ulceration
		Ischemic gangrene	4	5	Ischemic gangrene

Adapted from PARC manuscript.

Some of these endpoints are more useful for IC and some CLI. Cardiovascular events are extremely important in both IC and CLI because in general, the PAD population is at high risk for cardiovascular events. For this reason, clinical events committees often distinguish two measures of survival when evaluating the safety and effectiveness of two treatments: all-cause mortality and cardiovascular mortality. When adjudicating other cardiovascular events, such as myocardial infarction and stroke, universal definitions have been widely published and should be measured and adjudicated when conducting clinical trials [10,11].

Functional capacity refers to the distance or time that patients with PAD can ambulate, and it is usually measured by serial treadmill testing to assess a change in exercise performance during a clinical trial. Since the objective of most therapeutics for patients with PAD is to improve ambulatory status, the choice of which measures of functional capacity to include in clinical trials is critically important. The most common metrics used are maximum walking distance (MWD), absolute claudication distance (ACD), peak walking time (PWT), pain-free walking distance (PFWD), pain-free walking time (PFWT), and claudication onset time (COT). In addition, 6-min walk time (6MWT), a measure that does not involve treadmill testing, has also been utilized to measure functional capacity. In 1999, the Transatlantic Conference published guidelines recommending endpoints for studies of patients with IC and since then most clinical trials have used some combination of the aforementioned functional endpoints [8]. Although no consensus exists regarding which measure(s) to use, these endpoints do represent reproducible, safe, inexpensive measures that correlate well with patient-reported outcomes and are often sensitive when determining a treatment effect.

QOL measurements are also important for patients with both IC and CLI. QOL can be assessed using a nonspecific QOL measures as well as with disease-specific QOL measures. General or nonspecific measures include surveys such as the Medical Outcomes Study Short Form-36 (SF-36) questionnaire [12]. The SF-36 assesses the overall physical and mental functioning of a patient according to eight health dimensions: general health; change in health over the previous year; physical functioning; social functioning; role limitations due to physical restrictions; role limitations due emotional restrictions; mental health; and bodily pain [13]. Another general QOL measure is the EuroQOL-5D [14]. Disease-specific QOL measures include the Vascular QOL questionnaire (measures activity, symptoms, pain, emotional and social functioning), Walking Impairment Questionnaire (measures ability to walk certain distances, speeds, and climbing stairs), and the Peripheral Artery Questionnaire (measures physical limitations, symptoms, social function, treatment satisfaction, and overall QOL) [15–17]. These disease-specific questionnaires were intentionally created for the PAD population and thus are better suited to detect treatment effects in smaller PAD study populations. Most studies use some combination of QOL surveys; however, there is no current consensus regarding which QOL measure to utilize.

Lower extremity amputation has long been used as a measure of effectiveness in clinical trials involving patients with PAD, particularly those with CLI. Although amputation may seem to be a straightforward endpoint, controversy exists in clinical trials about how amputations are defined and counted. In particular, amputation is typically divided into major amputation and minor amputation. A major amputation is defined as any procedure that results in amputation at the level of the ankle or above, and is further divided on the basis of its location in relation to the knee. Below knee amputation is an amputation affecting the tibia at any point below the knee and above the ankle. Above knee amputation is an amputation above the knee, affecting the femur at any level. A minor amputation is defined as any procedure that results in amputation below the ankle, including the foot or toe(s). Although it is imperative to measure and/or adjudicate major and minor amputations in clinical trials, the impact of amputation when compared with other endpoints such as mortality, MI, stroke, and other limb-specific endpoints remains controversial [18–29].

Other limb-specific endpoints including acute limb ischemia, wound healing, analog pain scale, and disease progression are also important measures for patients with PAD. Acute limb ischemia is defined as a clinical history suggestive of a rapid decrease in limb perfusion and either a new pulse deficit with associated rest pain, pallor, paresthesia, or paralysis. Clinical trials often require confirmation of arterial thrombosis or thromboembolism by imaging, surgical findings, or pathological review [30]. When acute limb ischemia is present, patients have a high morbidity (including myocardial infarction, amputation, and loss of ambulatory status) and mortality.

Although preservation of the limb (ie, amputation prevention) is often a primary endpoint in clinical trials of patients with CLI, the use of endpoints such as wound healing and analog pain scale remains important. Wound healing is a subjective measurement in many cases since patients often present with wounds of different size/depth, different stages of healing before a clinical trial therapy has been initiated, and variable, alternative treatments such as wound care and hyperbaric oxygen therapy. In an attempt to more objectively measure wound healing, it should be recorded in a time-dependent manner such as time to complete wound healing. Analog pain scale measurements have been used more frequently for patients with CLI, and are fraught with bias and error due to how data is collected, a patient's individual perception of pain, and the interaction of other treatments such as narcotic analgesics.

In patients with PAD, disease progression is commonly measured using the following variables:

- Progression of PAD according to Rutherford or Fontaine classification
- Development of gangrene or a lower extremity necrotic wound or increasing size of an existing wound
- Hospitalization for IC, rest pain, ischemic ulcer (including debridement, antibiotic treatment or hydration for imaging)
- Hospitalization for lower extremity revascularization

Although these are broad categories, it is important to distinguish disease progression from clinical endpoints and safety events that occur during the process of clinical trials. Although not considered clinical endpoints or disease progression, another limb-specific measure, vessel patency, has often been measured in clinical trials of novel therapeutics for PAD, particularly devices. Vessel patency is further characterized into primary patency, primary assisted patency, and secondary patency. Primary patency is defined as uninterrupted patency following the procedure being evaluated. Primary-assisted patency is defined as vessel patency following a revision to prevent impending disease progression or stenosis. Secondary patency is defined as vessel patency after a repeat revascularization of an occluded artery.

Amputation-free survival (AFS) is a commonly employed composite endpoint in PAD studies, specifically in trials of patients with CLI. AFS is measured as the lack of either death or major amputation after a treatment assignment. Although AFS incorporates two valid and important endpoints as a combination endpoint, it weighs both a cardiovascular endpoint (death) and a limb-specific endpoint (major amputation) similarly, an issue that has been hotly debated in the vascular community over the past few years [31]. Depending on the therapeutic being tested, it may not be biologically plausible to affect both endpoints, thus reducing the statistical probability that a clinical trial meets its primary objective.

REVIEW OF PRIOR STUDIES

Many of the recommended cardioprotective medical therapies used in the PAD population work by preventing atherothrombotic events. These include statins, antiplatelets, and angiotensin-converting enzyme inhibitors. However, most of the data supporting their use in the PAD population has come from subgroup analyses in studies designed to evaluate patients with coronary and cerebrovascular disease rather than studies designed specifically to evaluate the PAD population [32–34]. Two examples of these trials include the Clopidogrel versus Aspirin in Patients at Risk of Ischemic Events (CAPRIE) [33] and the Heart Protection Study (HPS) [34], both of which generally demonstrated that cardiovascular mortality in the PAD population decreases similarly to the non-PAD population in response to these cardioprotective medications. These conclusions have both been further solidified in a more recent systematic review [35]. Although compelling, these conclusions are still based on data from subgroup analyses and there is a need for trials in the PAD-specific population as none currently exist.

IC

Heterogeneity in functional endpoints, single-arm observational study design, and poor subgroup reporting have all significantly limited the ability to compare effectiveness of therapies for PAD in clinical studies and meta-analyses. To date, evidence-based guidelines derived from metaanalyses such as the NICE (National Institute for Health and Care Excellence) guidelines have been limited in the number of studies to include in their analyses because they have focused on direct comparisons of specific therapies which are few and far between in the IC literature [36]. Studies report differing functional endpoints such as MWD, MWT, ACD, and PWT. QOL measures include at least five different instruments, most commonly SF-36 which is not a disease-specific measure. A few examples of such trials are discussed subsequently.

The CLEVER trial is a multicenter, randomized study that enrolled 111 patients with IC [37]. Patients were randomized to three arms: optimal medical care, optimal medical care plus supervised exercise, or optimized medical care plus endovascular revascularization. The primary endpoint was change in PWT at 6 months. There was a significant increase in the primary endpoint in the supervised exercise group when compared to the other two groups and in the endovascular revascularization group compared to the optimal medical therapy group. Secondary endpoints included free-living daily activity levels using pedometer readings, health-related QOL, and markers of cardiovascular health such as waist circumference, blood pressure, pulse pressure, resting pulse, c reactive protein, hemoglobin A1C, and lipids. There was a significant increase in QOL for those with supervised exercise. There was a trend toward a benefit with supervised exercise in the cardiovascular-health markers, but not significantly so. Although heralded as a pivotal clinical trial in the PAD field, the study struggled to enroll patients and enrollment in a fourth treatment group (supervised exercise plus endovascular revascularization) was terminated after eight patients were enrolled.

The RAVE trial looked at VEGF gene therapy with the primary endpoint of PWT at 12 weeks [38]. Secondary endpoints included ankle–brachial index, claudication onset time, and quality-of-life measures. The TRAFFIC trial investigated the use of recombinant fibroblast growth factor with the primary endpoint of PWT [39]. Secondary endpoints included ankle–brachial pressure index and safety. Although the primary efficacy endpoint was PWT in each of the aforementioned studies, the time points were different and the key secondary endpoints often differed, thus making it very difficult to compare treatment modalities across studies.

CLI

There are no approved disease-modifying medical therapies for treatment of CLI, thus the mainstay of treatment includes endovascular and surgical revascularization, of which it is not clear which is more efficacious [4]. With the lack of randomized controlled trials, the decision to attempt revascularization has largely been dependent on physician preference, patient preference, severity of symptoms, and anatomic considerations [18,40]. The objective performance goals discussed in this chapter are currently being established to attempt to standardize clinical outcome metrics in order to assist trial design for much needed studies investigating CLI [41].

Similar to IC research, CLI studies have also had much variation regarding endpoints assessed. In a recent analysis of 23 studies, few were found that assessed functional outcomes, QOL, and cardiovascular outcomes (MI, stroke) [4]. This same analysis also highlighted the fact that few studies directly compared endovascular treatment with surgical treatment, rather they compared two different surgical treatments or two different endovascular treatments. A few of the trials will be discussed subsequently, focusing on their endpoints.

The BASIL trial is the only randomized controlled CLI study comparing surgery to endovascular repair and it is now more than 10 years old [18]. Its primary endpoint was AFS at 6 months. Secondary endpoints include cost and health-related QOL. Although ultimately a negative study, the PREVENT III trial looked at E2F decoy therapy (edifoligide) in vein graft treatment with the primary endpoint of either graft reintervention or major amputation [40]. Secondary endpoints included all-cause graft failure, clinically significant graft stenosis, amputation/reintervention-free survival, and nontechnical primary graft patency.

The TAMARIS trial looked at fibroblast growth factor in patients with CLI deemed unsuitable for revascularization with the primary endpoint of time to major amputation or death [42]. There was no difference in the treatment group with respect to the primary endpoint. The TALISMAN trial (the Phase 2 preceding the TAMARIS trial) showed that the same fibroblast growth factor lead to significant reduction in major amputation and death at 1 year [43]. This disparity between results from Phase 2 to Phase 3 clinical trials likely resulted from differences in endpoints and other issues regarding the rigor of clinical trials (ie, blinding, follow-up).

ISSUES WITH ENDPOINTS

Given that there is not a current consensus on which endpoints are most useful and relevant, there is a great deal of variation in endpoints among individual studies and the way in which the endpoints are captured. This makes it extremely difficult to place individual studies into context when thinking of the entire PAD landscape. In addition, and perhaps more troublesome, given the heterogeneity in endpoints used, it is nearly impossible to effectively compare across studies and create practice changing conclusions that are meaningful and impact treatment decisions with everyday patients.

Another separate difficulty regarding more basic PAD research is that there is not an effective and predictable biological marker of PAD that can help guide early phase studies. This makes it extremely difficult to discern which early phase studies show promise and should be attempted in larger more time/cost intensive trials.

ANALYSIS OF OUTCOMES

As mentioned earlier, there is significant heterogeneity in the analysis of clinical trial results and this can drastically affect the outcome and interpretation of studies. For example, many CLI trials use a time-to-event analysis and composite endpoints. Time-to-event analyses are imperfect, as they do not capture repeat events that are particularly important in complex medical patients such as those with CLI. For example, in a time-to-event analysis of a composite endpoints that includes repeat revascularization, lower extremity amputation, and death, if a patient in a study has a repeat revascularization and then goes on to get an amputation and die; only the repeat revascularization will be counted as an endpoint and the amputation/death will be censored. In this example, a patient who died would be equivalent to a patient who just needed a repeat revascularization. In addition, nonfatal recurrent events are often frequent in CLI patients and the impact of these recurrent events is minimized by time-to-event analyses. Also, each composite endpoint is weighted similarly in a composite analysis, which is not clinically relevant as each individual endpoint in the composite analysis may mean very different things to both the patient and the clinician caring for the patient. Despite the potential limitations and pitfalls of composite endpoints, trials of PAD patients generally have a small sample size and the inclusion of a composite endpoint often is required when attempting to demonstrate a statistically significant result.

One potential solution to the composite endpoint dilemma and time-to-event analysis issues described previously is to implement a global rank method. This allows incorporation of recurrent events, differentiates the severity of events by assigning relative rankings to them, and permits different directionality of the effect of therapies on the composite endpoints [44]. This type of analysis was first proposed in 1984 and, despite early interest in its use in cardiovascular trials, it was not widely adopted because of a lack of expert consensus opinion regarding the relative ranking of endpoints [45]. Recently, the most important composite endpoints for CLI have been discussed and published in an attempt to guide future clinical trials (nine safety and efficacy standards including wound healing, rest pain, and repeat revascularization) [5]. This publication proposed a potential hierarchy of endpoints for CLI, namely (in descending order of severity): (1) death; (2) major amputation; (3) minor amputation; (4) incomplete wound healing; (5) complete wound healing; (6) complete pain resolution [31]. Although not perfect by any means, this represents a framework for moving forward in an attempt to gain a consensus for how to count and rank clinical endpoints for CLI studies.

Therapeutic benchmark controls (objective performance controls) have been frequently used in PAD studies as they allow single-arm studies and often permit a smaller sample size. The use of objective performance controls has been popular for device trials and the US Food and Drug Administration has permitted their use in pivotal studies, including Investigational Device Exemption studies used to obtain premarket approval (PMA). Although frequently used in patients with CLI, caution is necessary due to the heterogeneity of CLI in terms of clinical presentation, disease severity, and expected outcomes. In addition, the demographics of the CLI population have been changing over time as the prevalence of diabetes mellitus increases, thus an established historical control group may not readily apply to a current study population. Therefore, trials designed with the use of objective performance controls should be scrutinized carefully and the data obtained from them should be used with caution.

Lastly, many PAD researchers have difficulty obtaining adequate safety data regarding treatment modalities because sample sizes are small and safety endpoints are not consistently captured. One potential solution to this would be to more clearly define safety endpoints of interest and consistently measure these in all PAD studies. This effort will require a consensus panel of vascular specialists (experts from vascular surgery, vascular medicine, cardiology, and radiology).

GROUP EFFORTS TO DEFINE ENDPOINTS

Multiple groups have recently attempted to define clinical symptoms/signs and clinical endpoints. Each of the entities was developed in response to the need for consensus guidelines in the PAD field. Each has its own individual strengths and weaknesses. The subsequent paragraphs summarize each group's efforts and the important findings.

Peripheral Academic Research Consortium (PARC): PARC was an interprofessional collaboration consisting of academic members of the original Academic Research Consortium group that successfully established consensus definitions for coronary stent thrombosis. PARC established symptom definitions benchmarked to the two mentioned classification systems. Table 8.1 shows the two traditional classification systems along with the PARC consensus definitions. Although not yet validated, it is the consensus of the members of PARC that this classification system will clarify ambiguity regarding baseline symptoms and change in these symptoms during clinical trials. PARC was specifically engaged in outcome definitions for device studies, but many of the consensus ideas can be applied to other therapies such as regenerative medicine (ie, gene or cell therapy). Improvement in ABI, ultrasound, or angiography can act as a surrogate endpoint for success after various treatments. Table 8.2 is an example from the PARC document that shows specific values for these hemodynamic and imaging modules over time for an invasive procedure to be considered successful. These time points were chosen to match stages of wound healing and device behavior, along with common points of patient contact following interventions. Something similar to this table could be developed, tailored, and implemented in studies of regenerative medicine. PARC also recommended the collection of a wide array of functional measures in addition to hemodynamic and imaging measurements to help classify patients pre- and posttreatment. The most commonly recommended functional measurements included PWT, COT, and the 6MWT (Table 8.3).

Society of Vascular Surgery (SVS): Rutherford originally proposed standards for endpoints to be used when conducting research regarding limb ischemia in 1986. These have been adapted over the years and updated most recently by Rutherford himself in 1997 [46]. This system uses numerical terms to describe symptoms (Table 8.1) and signs of ischemia. These include walking distance

TABLE 8.2 Hemodynamic and Imaging Surrogate Endpoints for Patients With LE PAD

Hemodynamic and imaging surrogate endpoints				
Intermittent claudication				
Measurement technique	**Time point of evaluation**			
	Subacute (72 h to 30 days)	**3 months**	**6 months**	**12 months**
ABI (or TBI) at rest [7,49]	Increase in resting ABI or TBI ≥ 0.10 from preprocedure value	Resting ABI or TBI ≥ 0.10 from preprocedure value	Resting ABI or TBI ≥ 0.10 from preprocedure value	Resting ABI or TBI ≥ 0.10 from preprocedure value
		Failure in follow-up defined as reduction in ABI or TBI by 0.10 or return to preprocedure value		
Duplex ultrasound [7]	≤50% Diameter stenosis as defined by peak systolic velocity index (ratio of intrastenotic peak systolic velocity to prestenotic velocity) < 2.4	≤50% Diameter stenosis as defined by peak systolic velocity index (ratio of intrastenotic peak systolic velocity to prestenotic velocity) < 2.4	≤50% Diameter stenosis as defined by peak systolic velocity index (ratio of intrastenotic peak systolic velocity to prestenotic velocity) < 2.4	≤50% Diameter stenosis as defined by peak systolic velocity index (ratio of intrastenotic peak systolic velocity to prestenotic velocity) < 2.4
CT/MR/ invasive angiography [1,7]	≤ 50% Diameter stenosis or ≤ 70% area stenosis	≤ 50% Diameter stenosis or ≤ 70% area stenosis	≤ 50% Diameter stenosis or ≤ 70% area stenosis	≤ 50% Diameter stenosis or ≤ 70% area stenosis

Adapted from PARC manuscript.

and acute lower extremity ischemia including tissue viability. The CLI population has been growing more complex over the years with increasing rates of diabetes mellitus and end-stage renal disease, thus making it more difficult to target endpoints and compare studies across the CLI spectrum (rest pain, ulceration, gangrene). In order to help improve meaningful analysis of clinical outcomes in patients with CLI, the SVS has recently developed the Wound Ischemia Foot Infection (WIfI) classification system [47]. This classification scheme takes into account three major factors: wound severity, ischemia grade, and infection grade (Table 8.4). This newer system attempts to define an overall

TABLE 8.3 Clinical Outcomes for Patients With LE PAD

Clinical outcomes			
Intermittent claudication			
Domain			
Walking/functional capacity definitions [1,6,50]	Peak walking time (s)	Claudication onset time (s)	6-min walk test (ft./m)
	Assessed using a graded treadmill protocol that records the greatest time of exercise achieved that is limited by maximally tolerated claudication pain	Assessed using a graded treadmill protocol that records the time during exercise at the onset of claudication pain. Defines a clinically relevant endpoint, and may be responsive to treatment effect	Assessed on an unobstructed course of 50 or 100 ft. Measures the maximal distance walked after 6 min regardless whether the patient stops to rest or not (rest periods are acceptable)
Quality of life (recommended assessment tools per the PARC consensus)	Walking Impairment Questionnaire (WIQ)	Peripheral Artery Questionnaire (PAQ)	
	A validated disease-specific assessment of patient-reported outcomes that quantify the patient's ability to walk defined distance, speed, and stairs.	A disease-specific health status questionnaire that quantifies patient's physical limitations, symptoms, social function, treatment satisfaction, and quality of life.	
Clinical assessments [6,51]	Change in symptom classification: Report the change in symptom classification based on PARC classification	Clinical failure: Need for major repeat revascularization or lower extremity amputation	

Critical limb ischemia			
Amputation Definitions [5,6,51,52]	Lower extremity amputation	Major amputation	Minor amputation
	Any procedure that results in the removal of bone and tissue from the lower extremity	Any procedure that results in an amputation at the level of the ankle or above • Below knee amputation—amputation affecting the tibia at any point below the knee and above the ankle Above knee amputation—amputation above the knee, affecting the femur at any level	Any procedure that results in an amputation below the ankle, including the foot or toe(s)
Clinical assessment [5,7,47]	Major adverse limb events (MALE)	Wound healing	Ischemic pain relief
	Above ankle amputation of the index limb or major repeat revascularization (new bypass graft, jump/interposition graft revision, or thrombectomy/thrombolysis)	Complete epithelialization of an ischemic wound of target limb persistent for at least 14 days	Improvement in (or relief of) pain of target limb or at least 2 weeks using visual analog scale

Adapted from PARC manuscript.

TABLE 8.4 Society for Vascular Surgery Lower Extremity Threatened Limb (SVS WIfI) Classification System

W: Wound/clinical category

Grade	Ulcer	Gangrene
0	No ulcer	No gangrene
Clinical description: ischemic rest pain (requires typical symptoms + ischemia grade 3); no wound.		
1	Small, shallow ulcer(s) on distal leg or foot; no exposed bone, unless limited to distal phalanx	No gangrene
Clinical description: minor tissue loss. Salvageable with simple digital amputation (1 or 2 digits) or skin coverage.		
2	Deeper ulcer with exposed bone, joint or tendon; generally not involving the heel; shallow heel ulcer, without calcaneal involvement	Gangrenous changes limited to digits
Clinical description: major tissue loss salvageable with multiple (≥3) digital amputations or standard transmetatarsal amputation ± skin coverage.		
3	Extensive, deep ulcer involving forefoot and/or midfoot; deep, full thickness heel ulcer ± calcaneal involvement	Extensive gangrene involving forefoot and/or midfoot; full thickness heel necrosis ± calcaneal involvement
Clinical description: extensive tissue loss salvageable only with a complex foot reconstruction or nontraditional TMA (Chopart or Lisfranc); flap coverage or complex wound management needed for large soft tissue defect		

I: Ischemia

Hemodynamics/perfusion: measure TP or $TcPO_2$ if ABI incompressible (>1.3)

Grade	ABI	Ankle systolic pressure	TP, $TcPO_2$
0	≥0.80	>100 mmHg	≥60 mmHg
1	0.6-0.79	70–100 mmHg	40–59 mmHg
2	0.4-0.59	50–70 mmHg	30–39 mmHg
3	≤0.39	<50 mmHg	<30 mmHg

ABI, Ankle-brachial index; *PVR,* pulse volume recording; *SPP,* skin perfusion pressure; *TP,* toe pressure; *$TcPO_2$,* transcutaneous oximetry.Patients with diabetes should have TP measurements. If arterial calcification precludes reliable ABI or TP measurements, ischemia should be documented by $TcPO_2$, SPP, or PVR. If TP and ABI measurements result in different grades, TP will be the primary determinant of ischemia grade.Flat or minimally pulsatile forefoot PVR = grade 3.

TABLE 8.4 Society for Vascular Surgery Lower Extremity Threatened Limb (SVS WIfI) Classification System (*cont.*)

fI: foot Infection

SVS grades 0 (none), 1 (mild), 2 (moderate), and 3 (severe: limb and/or life-threatening). SVS adaptation of Infectious Diseases Society of America (*IDSA*) and International Working Group on the Diabetic Foot (IWGDF) perfusion, extent/size, depth/tissue loss, infection, sensation (*PEDIS*) classifications of diabetic foot infection

Clinical manifestation of infection	SVS	IDSA/PEDIS infection severity
No symptoms or signs of infection	0	Uninfected
Infection present, as defined by the presence of at least 2 of the following items: • Local swelling or induration • Erythema >0.5 to ≤2 cm around the ulcer • Local tenderness or pain • Local warmth • Purulent discharge (thick, opaque to white, or sanguineous secretion)	1	Mild
Local infection involving only the skin and the subcutaneous tissue (without involvement of deeper tissues and without systemic signs as described below). Exclude other causes of an inflammatory response of the skin (eg, trauma, gout, acute Charcot neuroosteoarthropathy, fracture, thrombosis, venous stasis)		
Local infection (as described previously) with erythema >2 cm, or involving structures deeper than skin and subcutaneous tissues (eg, abscess, osteomyelitis, septic arthritis, fasciitis), and no systemic inflammatory response signs (as described subsequently)	2	Moderate
Local infection (as described previously) with the signs of SIRS, as manifested by two or more of the following: • Temperature >38°C or <36°C • Heart rate >90 beats/min • Respiratory rate >20 breaths/min or $PaCO_2$ <32 mmHg • White blood cell count >12,000 or <4000 mm^3 or 10% immature (band) forms	3	Severe[a]

$PACO_2$, Partial pressure of arterial carbon dioxide; *SIRS*, systemic inflammatory response syndrome.
[a]*Ischemia may complicate and increase the severity of any infection. Systemic infection may sometimes manifest with other clinical findings, such as hypotension, confusion, vomiting, or evidence of metabolic disturbances, such as acidosis, severe hyperglycemia, new-onset azotemia.*
Adapted from SVS WIfI manuscript.

disease complexity/burden and more precisely ranks CLI severity in order to more accurately compare different patient groups at baseline and after treatment initiation. If WIfI continues to be utilized in future clinical studies, it will allow CLI patients to be more accurately compared across studies as well.

Trans-Atlantic Inter-Society Consensus for the Management of Peripheral Arterial Disease (TASC II): The last such consensus effort that will be mentioned in this chapter is the TASC II [48]. This group was created in order to help define diagnosis, treatment, and outcome measures not only for vascular specialists but also primary providers that encounter patients with PAD. The first edition of these guidelines emerged in 1999 and while broadly classifying functional endpoints for patients with PAD, its most common use has been in the definition and classification of lower extremity anatomic stenosis. This classification system defines lesions as either A, B, C, or D on the basis of the overall success rate of treating the lesion with surgical or endovascular techniques. Although useful to define a target lesion for treatment, TASC is limited in its overall applicability since many patients have lesions at more than one level [eg, inflow (aorto-iliac) and outflow (femoral-popliteal) stenosis].

PATH FORWARD

The path forward is not an easy one, nor is the correct answer absolutely clear at this point. What is clear is that the field of PAD remains significantly behind that of coronary artery disease and acute coronary syndrome, not only in the development of consensus endpoint definitions but also in the consistent use of consensus endpoints and in the number and breadth of clinical trials. Hope remains that groups such as PARC, SVS, and TASC continue to push for consistent application of inclusion/exclusion criteria, collection of clinical endpoints, and reporting of clinical endpoints in future clinical trials. As these endpoints are developed and validated, they must remain meaningful to all involved parties (patients, providers, and regulatory agencies). In general, both CLI and IC trials should report cardiovascular endpoints including cardiovascular mortality and/or all-cause mortality, MI, and stroke. Functional measures such as MWD, PWT, and 6MW should be measured and reported in all studies of IC patients, and amputation, wound healing, and analog pain scale should be measured and reported in all studies of CLI patients. Additionally, studies should report general QOL endpoints (SF-12 or SF-36) and/or disease-specific QOL endpoints such as the Walking Impairment Questionnaire or the Peripheral Artery Questionnaire. Although reporting all of these endpoints consistently may be somewhat cumbersome, it is the only way to make advances in research and improve the care for the PAD population. Although these endpoints may continue to evolve over the years, building on consensus definitions (as set forth by PARC, SVS, and TASC) will continue to solidify PAD research in years to come. This effort will require cooperation and interplay among PAD researchers, a diverse group of clinicians and clinical scientists, who have dedicated their lives to helping patients with PAD and will continue to strive to make these lofty goals come to full fruition.

CONCLUSIONS

Adapting a standard set of definitions for baseline symptoms, imaging/physiologic characterization and clinical outcomes/endpoints in PAD patients in ongoing and future clinical trials are crucial steps to conducting the most efficient and highest quality clinical research. The ability to effectively compare patients' baseline characteristics and outcomes between trials will accelerate regulatory approval and practice guideline development for emerging therapies. PARC, TASC, and SVS have developed some consensus definitions that form the base of a clinical trial foundation. Although the field of PAD research has much room for improvement, the concepts introduced in this chapter should be rapidly implemented in clinical trial methodology so that we continue to move the field forward.

REFERENCES

[1] Rooke TW, et al. 2011 ACCF/AHA focused update of the guideline for the management of patients with peripheral artery disease (updating the 2005 guideline): a report of the American College of Cardiology Foundation/American Heart Association Task Force on Practice Guidelines. J Am Coll Cardiol 2011;58:2020–45.

[2] European Stroke O, et al. ESC Guidelines on the diagnosis and treatment of peripheral artery diseases: Document covering atherosclerotic disease of extracranial carotid and vertebral, mesenteric, renal, upper and lower extremity arteries: the Task Force on the Diagnosis and Treatment of Peripheral Artery Diseases of the European Society of Cardiology (ESC). Eur Heart J 2011;32:2851–906.

[3] Jaff MR, Cahill KE, Yu AP, Birnbaum HG, Engelhart LM. Clinical outcomes and medical care costs among medicare beneficiaries receiving therapy for peripheral arterial disease. Ann Vasc Surg 2010;24:577–87.

[4] Jones WS, et al. Comparative effectiveness of endovascular and surgical revascularization for patients with peripheral artery disease and critical limb ischemia: systematic review of revascularization in critical limb ischemia. Am Heart J 2014;167:489–98.

[5] Conte MS, et al. Suggested objective performance goals and clinical trial design for evaluating catheter-based treatment of critical limb ischemia. J Vasc Surg 2009;50:1462–73.

[6] Creager MA, et al. ACCF/AHA/ACR/SCAI/SIR/STS/SVM/SVN/SVS Key data elements and definitions for peripheral atherosclerotic vascular disease: a report of the American College of Cardiology Foundation/American Heart Association Task Force on Clinical Data Standards (Writing Committee to develop Clinical Data Standards for peripheral atherosclerotic vascular disease). J Am Coll Cardiol 2012;59:294–357.

[7] Diehm N, et al. Clinical endpoints in peripheral endovascular revascularization trials: a case for standardized definitions. Eur J Vasc Endovasc Surg 2008;36:409–19.

[8] Labs KH, Dormandy JA, Jaeger KA, Stuerzebecher CS, Hiatt WR. Transatlantic Conference on Clinical Trial Guidelines in Peripheral Arterial Disease: clinical trial methodology. Basel PAD Clinical Trial Methodology Group. Circulation 1999;100:e75–81.

[9] Abbott JD. Lessons learned from recent randomized clinical trials for intermittent claudication. Circulation 2012;5:139–41.

[10] Leonardi S, et al. A novel approach to systematically implement the universal definition of myocardial infarction: insights from the CHAMPION PLATFORM trial. Heart 2013;99:1282–7.

[11] Thygesen K, et al. Third universal definition of myocardial infarction. J Am Coll Cardiol 2012;60:1581–98.

[12] Ware JE Jr, Sherbourne CD. The MOS 36-item short-form health survey (SF-36). I. Conceptual framework and item selection. Med Care 1992;30:473–83.

[13] Spronk S, et al. Intermittent claudication: clinical effectiveness of endovascular revascularization versus supervised hospital-based exercise training--randomized controlled trial. Radiology 2009;250:586–95.

[14] Dolan P. Modeling valuations for EuroQol health states. Med Care 1997;35:1095–108.

[15] McDermott MM, et al. Measurement of walking endurance and walking velocity with questionnaire: validation of the walking impairment questionnaire in men and women with peripheral arterial disease. J Vasc Surg 1998;28:1072–81.

[16] Morgan MB, Crayford T, Murrin B, Fraser SC. Developing the Vascular Quality of Life Questionnaire: a new disease-specific quality of life measure for use in lower limb ischemia. J Vasc Surg 2001;33:679–87.

[17] Spertus J, Jones P, Poler S, Rocha-Singh K. The peripheral artery questionnaire: a new disease-specific health status measure for patients with peripheral arterial disease. Am Heart J 2004;147:301–8.

[18] Adam DJ, et al. Bypass versus angioplasty in severe ischaemia of the leg (BASIL): multicentre, randomised controlled trial. Lancet 2005;366:1925–34.

[19] Duda SH, et al. Sirolimus-eluting versus bare nitinol stent for obstructive superficial femoral artery disease: the SIROCCO II trial. J Vasc Interv Radiol 2005;16:331–8.

[20] Duda SH, et al. Sirolimus-eluting stents for the treatment of obstructive superficial femoral artery disease: six-month results. Circulation 2002;106:1505–9.

[21] Fowkes F, Leng GC. Bypass surgery for chronic lower limb ischaemia. Cochrane Database Syst Rev 2008;16(2). CD002000.

[22] Green RM, et al. Prosthetic above-knee femoropopliteal bypass grafting: five-year results of a randomized trial. J Vasc Surg 2000;31:417–25.

[23] Kedora J, et al. Randomized comparison of percutaneous Viabahn stent grafts vs prosthetic femoral-popliteal bypass in the treatment of superficial femoral arterial occlusive disease. J Vasc Surg 2007;45:10–6. discussion 16.

[24] Krankenberg H, et al. Nitinol stent implantation versus percutaneous transluminal angioplasty in superficial femoral artery lesions up to 10 cm in length: the femoral artery stenting trial (FAST). Circulation 2007;116:285–92.

[25] Saxon RR, Dake MD, Volgelzang RL, Katzen BT, Becker GJ. Randomized, multicenter study comparing expanded polytetrafluoroethylene-covered endoprosthesis placement with percutaneous transluminal angioplasty in the treatment of superficial femoral artery occlusive disease. J Vasc Interv Radiol 2008;19:823–32.

[26] Schillinger M, et al. Sustained benefit at 2 years of primary femoropopliteal stenting compared with balloon angioplasty with optional stenting. Circulation 2007;115:2745–9.

[27] Schillinger M, et al. Balloon angioplasty versus implantation of nitinol stents in the superficial femoral artery. N Engl J Med 2006;354:1879–88.

[28] Sultan S, Hynes N. Five-year Irish trial of CLI patients with TASC II type C/D lesions undergoing subintimal angioplasty or bypass surgery based on plaque echolucency. J Endovasc Ther 2009;16:270–83.

[29] Twine CP, Coulston J, Shandall A, McLain AD. Angioplasty versus stenting for superficial femoral artery lesions. Cochrane Database Syst Rev 2009;15(2):CD006767.

[30] Bonaca MP, et al. Vorapaxar in patients with peripheral artery disease: results from TRA2{degrees}P-TIMI 50. Circulation 2013;127:1522–9.

[31] Subherwal S, et al. Use of alternative methodologies for evaluation of composite end points in trials of therapies for critical limb ischemia. Am Heart J 2012;164:277–84.

[32] Berger JS, Hiatt WR. Medical therapy in peripheral artery disease. Circulation 2012; 126:491–500.

[33] Committee CS. A randomised, blinded, trial of clopidogrel versus aspirin in patients at risk of ischaemic events (CAPRIE). CAPRIE Steering Committee. Lancet 1996;348:1329–39.

[34] Heart Protection Study Collaborative, G. MRC/BHF Heart Protection Study of cholesterol lowering with simvastatin in 20,536 high-risk individuals: a randomised placebo-controlled trial. Lancet 360, 7–22.

[35] Schmit K, et al. Comparative effectiveness review of antiplatelet agents in peripheral artery disease. J Am Heart Assoc 2014;3(6):e001330.

[36] Layden J, Michaels J, Bermingham S, Higgins B, Guideline Development G. Diagnosis and management of lower limb peripheral arterial disease: summary of NICE guidance. BMJ 2012;345:e4947.

[37] Murphy TP, et al. Supervised exercise versus primary stenting for claudication resulting from aortoiliac peripheral artery disease: six-month outcomes from the claudication: exercise versus endoluminal revascularization (CLEVER) study. Circulation 2012;125:130–9.

[38] Rajagopalan S, et al. Regional angiogenesis with vascular endothelial growth factor in peripheral arterial disease: a phase II randomized, double-blind, controlled study of adenoviral delivery of vascular endothelial growth factor 121 in patients with disabling intermittent claudication. Circulation 2003;108:1933–8.

[39] Lederman RJ, et al. Therapeutic angiogenesis with recombinant fibroblast growth factor-2 for intermittent claudication (the TRAFFIC study): a randomised trial. Lancet 2002; 359:2053–8.

[40] Conte MS, et al. Results of PREVENT III: a multicenter, randomized trial of edifoligide for the prevention of vein graft failure in lower extremity bypass surgery. J Vasc Surg 2006;43:742–51. discussion 751.

[41] Goodney PP, et al. Validation of the Society for Vascular Surgery's objective performance goals for critical limb ischemia in everyday vascular surgery practice. J Vasc Surg 2011;54:100–8.

[42] Belch J, et al. Effect of fibroblast growth factor NV1FGF on amputation and death: a randomised placebo-controlled trial of gene therapy in critical limb ischaemia. Lancet 2011;377:1929–37.

[43] Nikol S, et al. Therapeutic angiogenesis with intramuscular NV1FGF improves amputation-free survival in patients with critical limb ischemia. Mol Ther 2008;16:972–8.

[44] O'Brien PC. Procedures for comparing samples with multiple endpoints. Biometrics 1984;40:1079–87.

[45] Califf RM, Harrelson-Woodlief L, Topol EJ. Left ventricular ejection fraction may not be useful as an end point of thrombolytic therapy comparative trials. Circulation 1990;82:1847–53.

[46] Rutherford RB, et al. Recommended standards for reports dealing with lower extremity ischemia: revised version. J Vasc Surg 1997;26:517–38.

[47] Mills JL Sr, et al. The Society for Vascular Surgery Lower Extremity Threatened Limb Classification System: risk stratification based on wound, ischemia, and foot infection (WIfI). J Vasc Surg 2014;59:220–34.

[48] Norgren L. et al. Inter-society consensus for the management of peripheral arterial disease (TASC II). J Vasc Surg 2007;Suppl S: S5–S67.

[49] Aboyans V, et al. Measurement and interpretation of the ankle-brachial index: a scientific statement from the American Heart Association. Circulation 2012;126:2890–909.

[50] Hiatt, W.R. et al. Atherosclerotic Peripheral Vascular Disease Symposium II: nomenclature for vascular diseases. Circulation 118, 2826–2829.

[51] Geraghty PJ, Matsumura JS, Conte MS. Premarket assessment of devices for treatment of critical limb ischemia: the role of Objective Performance Criteria and Goals. J Vasc Surg 2009;50:1459–61.

[52] Bradbury AW, Investigators, B.t., & Participants. Bypass versus Angioplasty in Severe Ischaemia of the Leg (BASIL) trial in perspective. J Vasc Surg 51, 1S–4S.

Chapter 9

Endpoint Assessment for Critical Limb Ischemia for Cellular Therapy

W. Marston, MD
University of North Carolina, School of Medicine, Division of Vascular Surgery, Department of Surgery, Chapel Hill, NC, United States

INTRODUCTION

A review of the published medical literature seeking effective therapies for patients afflicted with critical limb ischemia (CLI) yields hundreds of articles elaborating on the benefits of a wide variety of treatments. These include herbal remedies, device therapies, growth factors, chelating agents, intermittent external limb pumps, hyperbaric oxygen therapy, cellular therapies, and many other options. The vast majority of these publications are little more than anecdotal cases, small treatment series, or preclinical studies establishing the potential benefit of promising novel agents. In order to craft rational treatment strategies for patients with this debilitating, limb-threatening disease, it is clear that systematic clinical studies are needed to carefully identify and document the benefits and risks each afford and in which patients. It is only through this mechanism that we can identify the truly beneficial therapies from those that, although theoretically useful, provide no actual clinical benefit to patients at high risk for limb loss.

Patients with CLI are often desperate for any hope to avoid amputation and will seek alternative therapies that may involve significant risk of complications with limited potential for improvement. Worse, they are also vulnerable to medical opportunists who may take advantage of their situation to convince patients to undergo "off label" or unapproved therapies at their own cost with unknown results. It is therefore imperative that potential CLI therapies are studied in well-defined protocols with outcome measures that are patient-focused and accurately reflect clinically meaningful improvement. For example, while an improvement in ankle–brachial index (ABI) may provide a signal that a therapy is achieving increased vascularization of a limb, this outcome is meaningless to the patient unless wound improvement, pain reduction, limb salvage, or another

Regenerative Medicine for Peripheral Artery Disease. http://dx.doi.org/10.1016/B978-0-12-801344-1.00009-7

patient-centered outcome occurs. In this chapter the potential clinical study endpoints will be reviewed along with their role in cellular therapy development.

CLI TREATMENT GOALS

The patient with CLI is faced with chronic rest pain of the affected limb (Rutherford Class 4), minor tissue loss (Class 5), or major tissue loss (Class 6). Although the most severe of the Class 6 patients may have a nonsalvageable limb, the remainder require treatment to reduce pain, heal open wounds, and preserve the limb or as much of it as is possible. In the event that limb salvage is not possible, the treatment goal then becomes healing of the amputated limb and rehabilitation to the highest level of function possible.

Balanced with the overall goal to achieve limb salvage is the realization that patients who present with symptomatic CLI have a limited life expectancy [1]. The median survival for these patients is less than 5 years [2]. Some subsets of CLI patients (particularly those with diabetes and renal failure requiring dialysis) have a life expectancy limited to less than a year. Therefore, treatment must consider options along with an assessment of the patient's life expectancy and the risks of any treatment under consideration. It is clear that the risk/benefit ratio of any CLI treatment should be well understood to incorporate it into the plan of care for this patient group.

For most patients, revascularization is the primary treatment option, either using a percutaneous endovascular approach or via surgical bypass. In the last 30 years an extensive catalog of device therapies has been developed to open arteries in the lower extremities affected by PAD. Balloon angioplasty and stenting were the initial therapies developed in the 1980s and 1990s [3]. Atherectomy, laser angioplasty, cryoplasty, drug-eluting balloons, and stents are a few of the more recent therapies employed to treat obstructed vessels in an effort to resupply the ischemic limb [4]. Surgical bypass is performed using autogenous vein or prosthetic materials such as polytetrafluoroethylene (PTFE) to bypass obstructed arteries in the limb. Unfortunately, despite the use of these methods, revascularization is occasionally not successful, or only partially successful in providing sufficient blood flow to the limb to relieve pain or heal ulcerated tissue [5]. Some patients have severe medical comorbidities that make them poor candidates for revascularization using any technique. In these cases, alternative therapies are considered.

Development of clinical studies of novel therapies for CLI requires assessment of a diverse set of characteristics depending on the primary goal of the individual study. Early phase clinical studies must focus primarily on safety outcomes relevant to CLI and the proposed therapy whereas later phase studies have the added goal of demonstrating efficacy. The study must be designed using outcomes that demonstrate safety and efficacy in a way that allows meaningful comparison to placebo or other CLI therapies without narrowing the inclusion criteria so much that the study outcomes are not reflective of the patients

TABLE 9.1 Endpoints in Critical Limb Ischemia (CLI) Trials

Clinical endpoints	
Amputation rate	Major amputation (above the ankle)
Time to amputation	Time to major amputation
Death	All-cause mortality
Amputation free survival (AFS)	Time to event: major amputation or death
Functional endpoints	
Rutherford or Fontaine class	Clinical classification of disease severity
Pain	As measured by Visual Analog Scale (VAS)
Quality of life (QoL)	As measured by SF-36 or VascuQol
Ulcer healing	Change in size or number of ulcers
Treadmill testing	Pain-free walking distance
Surrogate endpoints	
Ankle–brachial index (ABI)	Ratio of ankle to brachial blood pressure
Transcutaneous oxygen pressure ($TcPO_2$)	Noninvasive estimate of arterial blood flow
Angiography	Radiographic demonstration of blood flow

encountered in routine practice. The proposed endpoints for the study must occur frequently enough and be modifiable by the therapy so that the study can be powered adequately to achieve statistical significance. For instance, if a study is designed and powered on the basis of an expected amputation rate of 30% in a group of CLI patients but the actual amputation rate experienced in the study control group is only 15%, the study is likely to fail as it will be underpowered to detect a significant difference even if the therapy under consideration is able to benefit CLI patients. A list of potential endpoints that have been used in CLI trials is provided in Table 9.1. In this chapter we will examine these and other potential CLLI endpoints and their role in current study design.

ENDPOINT ASSESSMENT OPTIONS

Amputation/Amputation-Free Survival

In general, the primary goal of treatment in CLI is to prevent limb loss. To assess the usefulness of this endpoint in a specific clinical study it is critical to understand the event rate of this endpoint in the population to be studied. Conventional thinking has suggested that without revascularization, the majority of patients with CLI would eventually require amputation, either below (BKA) or above (AKA) the knee. It has therefore been concluded that a treatment modality that yielded a limb preservation rate of 80–90% would represent a clear improvement in the care of this patient population [3,4].

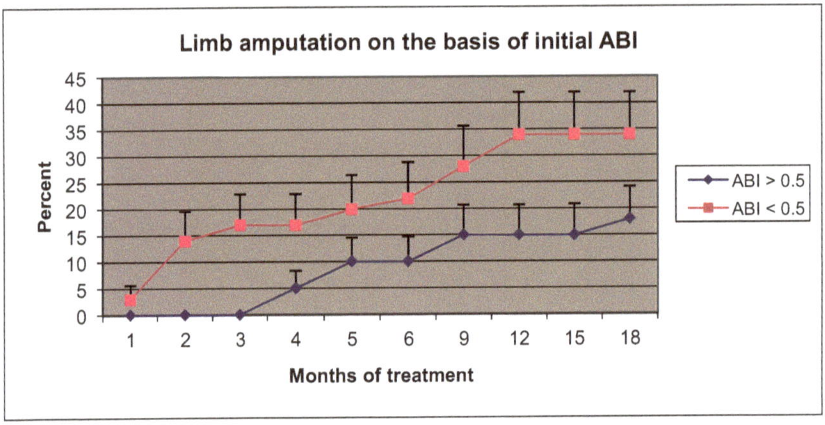

Months	0	3	6	12	18
Number of patients ABI > 0.5	51	49	40	33	32
Number of patients ABI < 0.5	39	34	31	24	23

FIGURE 9.1 **Incidence of limb amputation in limbs with an ABI > 0.5.**

However, more recent studies of the natural history of patients with CLI indicates that the limb loss rate in these patients, using the current accepted TransAtlantic Intersocietal Consensus (TASC) definition of CLI (ankle pressure < 70 mmHg, toe pressure < 50 mmHg), may be lower than previously believed. Marston et al. published a review of 169 patients with PAD and nonhealing wounds who were not candidates for revascularization or who chose conservative wound care rather than revascularization [6]. In the group with hemodynamic criteria of CLI, limb loss occurred in 38% at 12 months indicating that limb preservation was possible in the majority of CLI patients with tissue loss at 1 year (Fig. 9.1). In another study of the natural history of patients with tissue loss and PAD, Elgzyri et al. reported on 602 patients with an ankle pressure < 80 mmHg or toe pressure < 45 mmHg providing information on both amputation and AFS [7]. At a median follow-up of 30 weeks, 50% of the cohort had healed their wounds either primarily or after a minor amputation. Major amputation was required in 17% and 33% died unhealed (AFS 50%).

Using the TASC criteria to enroll patients with CLI for clinical trials of potential CLI therapies has resulted in surprisingly low amputation rates in control groups. It is possible that the most severely ischemic patients in the CLI group are screened out by the inclusion and exclusion criteria for studies of novel therapeutic agents. Most clinical studies exclude patients who, in the judgment of the investigator, are not likely to live for at least a year due to the follow-up requirements of the study. Other common exclusion criteria screening out CLI patients at the highest risk of limb loss or death include the

TABLE 9.2 Published 1-Year Event Rates From NO-CLI Trials

Author	Trial	Year	No.	Amp (%)	Death (%)	AFS (%)
Jivegard	Spinal cord stimulation	1995	26	50.0	30.8	X
Lepantalo	Retrospective clinical review	1996	105	46.3	54.3	28.0
Claeys	Spinal cord stimulation	1996	41	19.5	29.3	X
Klomp	Spinal cord stimulation	1999	60	48.3	23.3	40.0
Spincemaille	Spinal cord stimulation	2000	18	50.0	27.8	X
Am arm	Spinal cord stimulation	2003	39	46.2	0.0	54.0
Marston	Wound care only	2006	86	38.4	0.0	61.6
Brass	CIRCULASE (PGEi analog)	2006	190	10.5	10.0	81.0
Nikol	TALISMAN (NV1FGF)	2008	56	33.9	23.2	48.2
Hiatt	TAMARIS (NV1FGF)	2010	259	21.2	15.1	66.8
Powell	Intramuscular hepatocyte GF	2010	6	33.3	16.7	X

AFS, Amputation-free survival; *Amp*, amputation; *GF*, growth factor; *NO-CLI*, no option critical limb ischemia; *NV1FGF*, nonviral 1 fibroblast growth factor; *PGE*, prostaglandin E; *X*, not documented.

exclusion of patients with severe renal insufficiency and those who have limited functional status.

The Circulase trial evaluated the use of lipo-ecrapost a PGE1 analog in limiting amputations [8]. The inclusion criteria required an ankle pressure less than 50 mmHG and TP less than 30 mmHG for patients with rest pain, and an ankle pressure less than 70 mmHG and TP less than 50 mmHG for tissue loss/gangrene. Despite the use of these strict criteria the 6-month amputation rate was only 13% in the placebo arm. In 2012, Benoit et al. reviewed amputation, death and AFS rates from 11 studies reporting these outcomes in patients with CLI not undergoing revascularization between 1995 and 2010 (Table 9.2) [9]. The authors observed that the overall incidence of amputation was 34% and the number remaining free of amputation or death (AFS) was 55%. More importantly, they found that there was evidence of improvement in these outcomes over time, with regression analysis indicating that AFS has risen over time as mortality rates improve. Considering only the five studies contributing data to their analysis published between 2006 and 2012, the amputation rate in the NO-CLI patient population was 21.6%, the death rate at a year was 14.1% and the amputation free survival rate was 70.1%.

To emphasize the critical impact these outcomes have on clinical trial design and successful execution, the example of the development of NV1FGF can be considered. NV1FGF is a plasmid-based angiogenic gene delivery system that was evaluated in several clinical trials for its affect on clinical outcomes in patients with CLI. After several growth factor trials failed to produce a sufficiently robust angiogenic response to improve outcomes in patients with CLI, it was postulated that the use of this gene delivery system would result in ongoing growth factor expression in the ischemic tissue of the leg resulting in a more robust angiogenic response. In the Talisman study, a Phase-II randomized placebo-controlled study of 125 patients with CLI, the incidence of amputation in the control group was 33.9% [10]. The NV!FGF treated limbs experienced a limb loss rate that was significantly lower at 15.7% ($p = .015$). AFS was 51.8% in the control group and 27.4% in the NV1FGF group ($p = .009$). On the basis of the results of this study a Phase-III trial was performed in 525 patients to confirm the efficacy of NV1FGF for patients with CLI [11]. However, the event of amputation in the control group in Phase-III (21.2%) was lower than the amputation rate in the Phase-II (33.9%). The amputation and AFS rates in the NV1FGF treated limbs were similar in the Phase-III study to the Phase-II study, but this was not significantly lower than the control group, yielding a failed primary outcome.

It is clear that the specific criteria used to select patients for CLI studies have a major impact on the event rate, even within the boundaries described by the TASC hemodynamic criteria for CLI. Vallabhaneni et al. examined the relationship between toe and ankle pressures and amputation/AFS rates in NO-CLI patients [12]. In a retrospective evaluation of 345 limbs treated without revascularization, the authors found that the overall limb loss was 24% at 1 year and in 31% at 3 years. Mortality was 32% at 1 year and 56% at 3 years. Amputation-free survival was 54% at 1 year and 28% at 3 years. In this patient population with a high incidence of DM and/or renal insufficiency, ankle pressures were frequently unobtainable due to severe calcification (62%). In most cases, toe pressures were relied on to qualify patients as being in the CLI category. They evaluated the relationship of a toe pressure between 0 and 50 to the rate of amputation. Lower toe pressures were associated with a significantly higher incidence of amputation. Among those with an initial toe pressure less than or equal to 10 mmHg ($n = 85$), limb loss occurred in 46 % at 1 year and 60% at 3 years. This incidence was significantly greater than limb loss among those with a toe pressure 31–50 mmHg (18% at 3 years, $p < .001$, Fig. 9.2). Amputation free survival also varied significantly on the basis of baseline toe pressure as noted in Table 9.3.

Risk Factors Related to Amputation and AFS

Rest Pain/Wound Healing

Within the CLI category of PAD, it has been reported that patients with rest pain have a significantly lower risk of amputation than patients with tissue loss. In the RESTORE-CLI trial studying the effect of Ixmyelocel-T cellular therapy on patients with CLI, there was a difference in the AFS for patients with rest pain (87.5%) compared to those with tissue loss (56%) [13]. In a study of

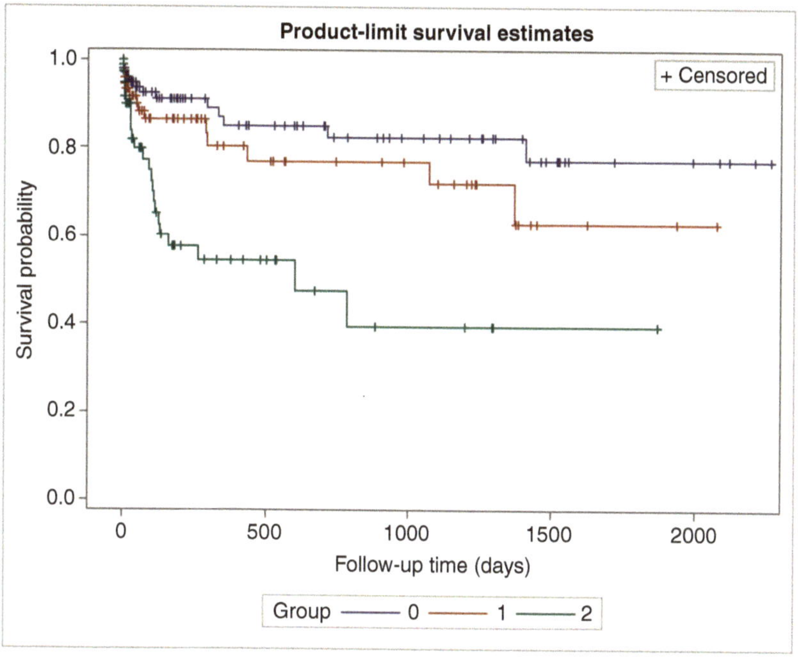

FIGURE 9.2 Incidence of limb preservation over time in nonrevascularized limbs separated by initial toe pressure. Follow-up time is in days. Group 0: Toe pressure 31–50 mmHg, $n = 115$; Group 1: Toe pressure 11–30 mmHg, $n = 82$; Group 2: Toe pressure 0–10 mmHg, $n = 85$; Survival probability = limb preservation.

TABLE 9.3 K-M Amputation-Free Survival by Revised Toe Hemodynamic Pressure Group, $n = 282$ limbs

	6 month	1 year	2 year	3 year
Overall	0.64 (0.031)	0.54 (0.032)	0.41 (0.033)	0.28 (0.032)
Toe pressure 31–50 (Group 0, $n = 115$)	0.82 (0.040)	0.71 (0.048)	0.58 (0.053)	0.44 (0.056)
Toe pressure 11–30 (Group 1, $n = 82$)	0.69 (0.054)	0.53 (0.060)	0.38 (0.060)	0.27 (0.057)
Toe pressure 0–10 (Group 2, $n = 85$)	0.36 (0.055)	0.35 (0.055)	0.21 (0.050)	0.08 (0.036)

In comparison to Group 0: Adjusted HR, Toe Hemodynamic Pressure Group 1: 1.66 (1.12,2.47), $p = 0.01$*;
Adjusted HR, Toe Hemodynamic Pressure Group 2: 3.25 (2.22,4.76), $p < 0.0001$*.

an autologous BM concentrate enrolling 48 patients presenting with rest pain (n = 18) or tissue loss (n = 30), Iafrati et al. reported that no amputations occurred in the Rutherford class 4 group compared to a limb loss rate of 33% in the Rutherford class 5 group [14]. They concluded that if a CLI study included a significant number of R4 patients, amputation or AFS would not be appropriate standalone outcome measures.

Endpoint Time Frame for Amputation

One clear problem with the use of amputation as a study endpoint for CLI trials relates to the lack of universally accepted objective criteria defining when amputation is necessary. Amputation is generally recommended if a patient has tissue necrosis or infection that is extensive such that excision of the necrotic/infected material would render the remaining limb inadequate for ambulation. This is a complex decision that varies depending on the patient's general medical status, the condition of the contralateral limb, their strength and balance. Also, the decision may be altered by the patient's interest and suitability to embark on a prolonged aggressive wound care treatment regimen that may require 6–12 months or more to achieve a healed wound. As a result, amputation may be appropriate for a patient with more limited forefoot involvement who would not be ambulatory with a transmetatarsal amputation due to contralateral limb loss or other reasons. However, in another patient, more extensive forefoot, midfoot, or even heel involvement may be appropriate to consider aggressive prolonged efforts at salvage.

The other primary reason to recommend amputation is for patients who have intractable ischemic rest pain with no option for revascularization. This is clearly a decision that is individualized on the basis of the patient's pain tolerance, the overall affect on quality of life and the risk of amputation. Patients will often delay amputation for months or even years despite severe ischemia and no option for improvement. In clinical trials, patients may delay amputation in the hope that the study treatment will improve their symptoms. This may continue through the primary endpoint timeframe and therefore these patients are counted in the limb preservation group despite chronic pain and poor QOL, which may lead to eventual amputation later.

On the basis of this information it is clear that using amputation and/or AFS as an endpoint in CLI patients yields a challenging dilemma for trial design. If the enrollment criteria are designed to eliminate the worst patients with the lowest hemodynamic criteria, or those with severe wounds, the patients are more likely to survive to complete the study protocol and the serious adverse events will be less frequent. However, the incident rate for amputation will be lower and may not leave sufficient room for the treatment under test to demonstrate a significant reduction in the amputation or AFS rate. Conversely, if the enrollment criteria are tuned to enroll the worst patients with the lowest pressures and tissue loss, the amputation and AFS rates will increase but the number of patients surviving long enough for meaningful endpoint analysis will decrease which may affect the power calculations significantly.

Choosing a relatively short endpoint timeframe of 3–6 months invokes the risk that patients who are not benefitted by their assigned treatment will tolerate their symptoms past the endpoint despite a lack of real improvement. Moving to an endpoint with a longer time frame of 12 or 24 months reduces the affect of patient tolerance on amputation but increases the time and cost of the study and the incidence of mortality in the patient population leading to fewer evaluable patients requiring a larger sample size.

Rest Pain

Improvement in rest pain is commonly captured as an endpoint for CLI studies. For R4 patients, pain is the primary symptom and the goal of any therapy is to relieve pain and improve QOL. The visual analog scale is a well-validated instrument to measure pain levels. It has been demonstrated to be responsive to intervention but is subject to relatively low repeatability as the day-to-day pain level for an individual patient is frequently variable based on a variety of factors. If the endpoint is measured at a specific time and does not average a series of assessments the true impact of a patients pain is not well captured. One option is to require subjects to maintain a diary of their pain level with frequent assessments to better characterize their average pain level.

Although many R5 patients also have significant rest pain, others do not feel ischemic rest pain due to the coexistence of neuropathy, particularly in patients with DM. R5 patients also may experience improvement in their rest pain during a study but may fail therapy due to wound specific problems, particularly recurrent infection that may lead to increased tissue loss and eventual amputation despite improved vascular supply [15].

Considering improvement in pain as the primary endpoint for a CLI study would lead to a limited patient group for enrollment, primarily R4 patients and well-selected R5 patients. Due to the subjective nature of this endpoint and its daily variability it is unclear whether pain improvement would be an acceptable endpoint for a CLI therapy seeking FDA approval if no other benefit such as limb preservation or QOL improvement was demonstrated.

Wound Healing

Wound healing is a meaningful outcome measure for patients with CLI. Many patients with CLI experience little rest pain due to peripheral neuropathy and present for medical care to wound specialists for management of a chronic nonhealing lower extremity ulcer. Persistence of a nonhealing ulcer places the patient at increased risk for wound infection, osteomyelitis, and potential progression to amputation. Wound healing is associated with improvement in QOL for this patient population compared to nonhealers. For Rutherford class 5 and

6 patients, ulcer healing with a functional foot is the primary goal, allowing the patient to resume activity and significantly reducing the risk of limb loss.

As an outcome measure, wound closure is relatively objective, although the exact appearance of a closed wound may be susceptible to individual interpretation. Photographic documentation may be used to confirm wound healing allowing review and confirmation by additional observers if desired. Wound healing occurs slowly if at all in patients with CLI. In a study of the natural history of patients with chronic nonhealing lower extremity ulcers and arterial insufficiency managed without revascularuzation, time to wound healing was measured [6]. At 1 year of follow-up, limb loss occurred in 25% of patients, 50% of wounds healed after a year of follow-up and 25% of patients still had a limb with an open wound after a year of chronic wound management.

Studies using wound healing as an outcome measure must determine how to address the inclusion of adjunctive therapies sometimes used in addition to standard care to heal wounds. Randomized clinical trials in nonischemic chronic wounds have validated the benefit of several of these adjunctive therapies. Two topical living cellular therapies, Dermagraft and Apligraf, have been approved by the FDA for use in diabetic foot ulcers with adequate vascular supply [16,17]. Platelet-derived growth factor (Becaplermin) was also found in randomized studies to increase the healing of DFUs [18]. Recently, several newer skin substitutes have been approved for use in chronic wounds including amniotic membrane constructs and other cellular and non-cellular therapies. None of these therapies have been tested adequately in patients with poor vascular supply and the product labeling of most specifically identifies that they are not indicated for wounds with significant arterial insufficiency. Given that these products are not designed for patients with CLI and have not been adequately tested to determine whether they provide benefit for this patient group, they should generally be excluded from use in studies using wound healing as a primary outcome measure.

A weakness of this outcome measure is that is not relevant in Rutherford class 4 patients who do not have open wounds. Standardization of care may be difficult due to the variety of options available for management of chronic wounds. In order to optimally care for patients with chronic nonhealing wounds, defined wound care programs with wound specialists are useful. Standard wound care at a high level requires expertise in methods of wound debridement, control of bacteria and treatment of infection, and offloading pressure from ulcers over bony prominences. In some situations, partnerships of vascular specialists and wound-care specialists are beneficial to provide optimal management in CLI protocols focused on wound healing.

Previous studies using wound healing as an endpoint have identified other difficulties with this measure. In the Talisman Phase-II study of NV1FGF, wound healing was employed as the primary efficacy outcome [10]. There was no significant improvement in ulcer healing identified in the study, even though the use of NV1FGF significantly reduced the incidence of major amputation.

The authors felt that this was in part due to the large variety of wounds enrolled in the study with excessive variation in wound size and tissue quality. In addition, wound care was not standardized across the investigational sites leading to significant variation in treatment methods.

A final consideration for studies evaluating wound healing as an outcome measure concerns the sites of drug administration. Typically, studies in patients with CLI have focused on administering therapy to the lower leg via intramuscular injections, typically in the calf. It is unclear whether an angiogenic therapy would have any benefit when administered remote to an ischemic wound that typically occurs on the foot or ankle. For this reason, consideration should be given to peri- or intrawound administration of treatments if the primary goal is wound closure.

Quality of Life

A variety of quality of life (QOL) measurement tools have been utilized in studies of PAD to define the affects on QOL and measure improvement after treatment. Generally it has been recommended that an assessment of general QOL such as the SF-36 be paired with a measure of disease-specific health such as the vascular quality of life (VascuQOL) or PAD quality of life (PADQOL) questionnaires. In general, disease specific patient-reported outcome measures (PROMs) in PAD are designed to measure the effect of claudication and rest pain on QOL and lack specific questions related to foot ulcers and their affect on the patient's QOL. In particular, the typical diabetic neuropathic patient with CLI may not experience severe pain but may have poor quality of life due to the need to avoid ambulation and wear heavy offloading footwear restricting mobility severely. These and other specific issues in the CLI population may not be well captured and the responsiveness to intervention of these measures may be limited when the goal is to heal tissue loss rather than to increase walking distance.

While there have been limited assessments of disease-specific PROMs In the CLI population, Sprangers et al. used the SF-36 to assess patients with no-option CLI, yielding scores below the general population mean on every assessment of the SF-36 [19]. The most severely affected scores were in the areas of physical functioning and bodily pain. Landry et al. used the SF-36 and VascuQOL scores to evaluate QOL improvement after revascularization in patients with CLI [20]. Using the SF-36, the only significant change in this assessment of general health after revascularization was a reduction in bodily pain. Using the VascuQOL, all measured parameters of this disease-specific measure improved significantly after successful revascularization.

Most studies in patients with CLI have not chosen a quality of life assessment score as a primary outcome measure. These are usually secondary outcomes, playing a supportive role to the primary outcome. Although patient QOL is an important outcome when treating any condition, the currently employed outcome scoring systems have limited evidence validating them as sensitive indicators of improvement after intervention in CLI patients. A recent review of the quality of the currently available disease specific patient reported outcome measures examined the VascuQol, PAD-QOL questionnaire, and several other QOL evaluations for accuracy, reproducibility and responsiveness to treatment [21]. Overall, it was found that evidence supporting the validity of these scoring systems was limited, leading to a lack of confidence in conclusions based on them. For these reasons they have not typically been accepted by regulatory agencies as key outcome measures in clinical trials of therapies for the treatment of CLI. With further development and validation, it is possible that this may change in the future.

Surrogate Outcome Measures

Most clinical trials select various surrogate outcome measures in CLI studies to probe for signals that the therapy under investigation is resulting in some measurable improvement. Increases in ABI, toe pressure, transcutaneous oxygen levels, and laser Doppler flowmetry results occurring after initiation of a therapy are suggestive of benefit. These findings are useful as they suggest some active measurable improvement in limb perfusion related to the study therapy. In practice, clinical markers for limb perfusion that measure blood pressure of the pedal vessels such as ABI or TP are difficult to increase consistently without revascularization of the limb. Strategies designed to stimulate regeneration of tissue may not increase distal blood flow sufficiently to increase intraluminal pressures, yet still have a positive affect on limb preservation, pain control and QOL.

Transcutaneous oxygen measurement (TCOM) and laser Doppler flowmetry are also frequently used measures of limb perfusion in patients with PAD. Both have been found to correlate with ABI and toe pressures but are less affected by vessel calcification making them attractive for use in patients with CLI [22]. In a study evaluating the use of intermittent pneumatic compression for patients with CLI, patients treated with IPC experienced an increase in transcutaneous PO_2 that was significantly greater than in the control group [23]. This increase in $TcPO_2$ was associated with significantly higher limb salvage rates. In a comparative study, Yamada et al. studied 211 patients with ischemic tissue loss using ABI, toe pressure, TCOM, and skin perfusion pressure (SPP) using laser Doppler [24]. Comparing the tests and their ability to predict wound healing, SPP was the most predictive test with a sensitivity of 72% and specificity of 88%. The best correlation using a combination of studies to predict wound healing was obtained using the SPP and toe pressure together (correlation with sound healing $r = 0.69$).

Unfortunately, both TCOM and laser Doppler tests are susceptible to variation depending on the specific testing protocols used and locations tested on the ischemic limb. Limb positioning, room temperature, and other variables may have a major affect on result reproducibility. Both modalities provide a measurement at a specific location on the lower extremity, such as the great toe, the dorsum of the foot, the plantar surface of the foot or ankle. Results may vary significantly between these locations making it difficult to determine how to use the information obtained from these studies as an outcome measure for clinical studies.

Other methods that may be considered for evaluation of the microcirculation of the lower extremity include indocyanine green angiography, hyperspectral imaging, and scanning laser Doppler. While these have demonstrated potential to identify changes in limb perfusion in response to intervention, they are primarily qualitative studies that do not have quantifiable results that have been documented in relation to wound healing, limb preservation, or other hard outcomes for patients with CLI.

In practice, cellular therapies for CLI have not consistently stimulated a significant increase in any of these measures of limb perfusion. It is thought that currently employed surrogate outcomes may not be sensitive enough to identify changes that are occurring, or that the mechanism of action of cellular therapy may not involve clinically perceptible changes in blood flow or oxygen delivery to the ischemic limb.

To date, surrogate outcome measures have not been accepted by the FDA as an outcome for approval of a cellular therapy for CLI. However, use of these modalities in clinical trials will continue as they can provide evidence of actual changes in limb perfusion or oxygenation that would support clinically meaningful outcomes if achieved during these trials.

Prevention of Need for Revascularization

To date, no clinical trials for patients with CLI have utilized avoidance of revascularization procedures as an outcome measure. For some patients, prevention of need for revascularization, either percutaneous or surgical, is an important goal. Revascularization involves risk of complication, pain and discomfort, recovery time and significant cost. Although the risk of complication and recovery time are significantly less with percutaneous methods of revascularization, there remain infrequent complications and both methods of revascularization are associated with significant cost to the health care system. CLI patients frequently have significant cardiac, pulmonary and renal comorbidities that affect their suitability for revascularization, either percutaneous or surgical. A therapy that reduces pain, prevents wound worsening and allows the patient to avoid revascularization may add significant value to the treatment pathway.

Composite Measures

Due to the difficulties in trial design and execution encountered using amputation, amputation-free survival, and some of the other outcome measures discussed, a number of investigators have turned to composite outcome measures. These strategies aim to combine several clinically meaningful outcomes into one aggregate outcome measure providing the advantage of increasing the incidence that one of the endpoints is reached. This allows a greater potential separation between treatment and control groups reducing the number needed to treat to potentially reach a significant endpoint.

There has been a concerted effort to define composite endpoints for the evaluation and comparison of revascularization procedures for CLI. The Society for Vascular Surgery developed objective performance goals (OPGs) for CLI using a composite endpoint, major adverse limb events (MALE) as one of their primary outcome measures [25]. This endpoint includes major amputation and major reintervention, defined as creation of a new surgical bypass, graft revision, thrombectomy or thrombolysis. The proposed OPG states that after revascularization patients should experience freedom from peri-operative death or MALE in 71% at 1 year of follow-up (Table 9.4). This and other OPGs were validated in a study of 1039 patients undergoing lower extremity revascularization at a broad selection of hospitals indicating the usefulness of this endpoint in the clinical practice of patients with CLI [26]. This data confirms the outcomes achieved both at centers of excellence and at community practices are comparable using MALE as an outcome measure. The authors conclude that it is reasonable to use this endpoint in revascularization studies as a target to compare novel device strategies and their suitability for clinical use.

Several limitations of the traditional use of composite endpoints must be considered. First, each of the components of the composite endpoint counts equally in the analysis, thus considering them to be of equal clinical significance. Although death or major amputation would be considered to the patient to be more important outcomes than need for revascularization, these would be statistically equally weighted using traditional composite endpoint analysis.

TABLE 9.4 Summary of Efficacy Outcomes (1 year) for Overall CLI Cohort and Suggested OPG for Each Endpoint

Outcome	Point (95% CI)	Efficacy OPG (%)
MALE + POD	76.9% (74.0–79.9)	71
AFS	76.5% (73.7–79.5)	71
RAS	46.5% (42.3–51.2)	39
RAO	61.3% (58.0–64.9)	55
Limb salvage	88.9% (86.7–91.1)	84
Survival	85.7% (83.3–88.1)	80

AFS, Amputation-free survival; *CI,* confidence interval; *CLI,* critical limb ischemia; *MALE,* major adverse limb event; *OPG,* objective performance goals; *POD,* perioperative death; *RAO,* any reintervention or above ankle amputation of the index limb; *RAS,* any reintervention, above ankle amputation of the index limb, or stenosis. Rates reported as proportion free from adverse event.

Also, only the first-occurring event in the composite is counted in traditional endpoint analysis, with any subsequent outcomes being ignored. In traditional analysis a patient who required revascularization, then amputation and died would be statistically no different from a patient who required revascularization then was alive with an intact limb.

To account for these limitations, Suberwhal et al. have proposed the use of alternative methodologies including the global rank method for analysis of composite end points in CLI trials [27]. Using this method, clinical investigators would agree prior to study initiation on a hierarchy of relevant endpoints based on their clinical importance. Optimally, this hierarchy should be based on a broad consensus including expert opinion, FDA input, insurer input and input from other stakeholders. Also, the criteria included in the ranking should be outcomes that the therapy under trial would be expected to affect. Patients suffering a worse outcome such as death receive a worse outcome than those suffering a less severe outcome such as need for revascularization and this is reflected in the statistical analysis. Using this analysis, a therapy would be required to have a larger affect on a less severe outcome to satisfy the endpoint than on a more severe outcome. Advantages of this study design is the ability to better characterize the variety of outcomes that occur in CLI patients, both in severity and frequency and to allow reduction in the number needed to enroll to achieve a meaningful endpoint. Disadvantages include potential difficulty in reaching agreement between stakeholders on the relative importance of various outcome measures in the global rank score, and the lack of generation of standard survival curves.

To date neither MALE nor composite endpoints using the global rand scoring method have been used in studies of CLI patients who are not good candidates for revascularization and would generally be the primary candidates for cellular therapy. It is possible that further consideration of these outcome measures would pave the way for FDA recognition of the utility of a meaningful composite endpoint for future studies.

Endpoint Assessment in Recent CLI Studies Using Cellular Therapy

Recently published cellular therapy studies with their identified endpoints are listed in Table 9.5. Given that most of these have been early phase clinical trials in Phase-I or dosing studies, the primary endpoint has most often been a safety assessment. In those that listed an efficacy endpoint as the primary, two employed major amputation at 120 days or 6 months [28,29]. One study identified ABI as the primary endpoint [30], and two chose a composite endpoint [13,31]. In one case the composite endpoint captured a time to treatment failure with amputation, death, doubling of wound size, or development of new gangrene comprising the definition of treatment failure [13]. In the other study employing a composite, the authors developed an efficacy score, representing changes in the toe brachial pressure index (TBPI), Wong–Baker FACES pain rating scale,

TABLE 9.5 Recently published cellular therapy studies in critical limb ischemia patients with their identified endpoints

Author	Year published	study	Phase	# patients	Primary endpoint	Secondary endpoints
Teraa [28]	2015	JUVENTAS trial		160	Major amputation at 6 months	Minor amputations, mortality, QOL, rest pain, ABI, $TcPO_2$
Iafrati [14]	2011	Harvest BM aspirate concentrate	Pilot	48	Safety	Amputation, pain, ABI, $TcPO_2$, QOL score, composite
Kawamoto [31]	2009	CD34+ cells	1/!!a	17	Composite efficacy score	Pain scale, $TcPO_2$, TBI, ulcer size, walking distance
Lasordo [32]	2013	CD34+ cells	Pilot	28	Safety	Amputation, time to amputation, pain, walking distance, QOL
Murphy [33]	2011	BM mononuclear	I	30	Safety	TBI, ABI, $TcPO_2$, pain, QOL, ulcer healing
Powell [13]	2012	Ixmyelocel-T	II	72	Composite time to treatment failure	AFS, amputation, wound size, safety
Gupta [34]	2013	BM-MSCs	I	20	Safety	ABI, rest pain, wound healing, amputation
Lu [35]	2010	BM-MSCs	Pilot	82	Safety	wound healing, walking time, ABI, $TcPO_2$, MRA
Prochazka [29]	2010	BM concentrate		96	Major amputation at 120 days	Pain, functional status, ABI, TBI, $TcPO_2$, SPP, laser Dopp
Walter [30]	2011	BM-MNC PROVASA	Pilot	40	ABI at 3 and 6 months	Wound healing, AFS, rest pain

and total walking distance 12 weeks after cell transplantation [31]. Of note, none of these studies were pivotal trials and thus their endpoints were more often exploratory rather than data expected to achieve FDA approval for market.

Two Phase-III studies of cellular therapy, initiated since 2010 were developed as pivotal trials to support applications for FDA approval in patients with CLI. The REVIVE trial was developed as a pivotal study evaluating the benefit of IM injections of Ixmyelocel-T expanded BM-mononuclear cells compared to placebo in patients with no options for revascularization. The primary endpoint was AFS at 12 months. Similarly, the pivotal study of the Harvest autologous BM concentrate system for CLI used AFS as the primary endpoint, but measured at 6 months. Both of these studies were eventually halted early due to inability to enroll a sufficient number of patients for analysis, likely due to the inclusion/exclusion criteria requiring that the patients have no option for revascularization. It is difficult to evaluate outcomes in 2 groups of patients using amputation or AFS as the endpoint if a large number of patients are revascularized after study enrollment. The revascularization creates the question of whether the outcomes are driven by the cellular therapy under consideration or the revascularization procedure.

Extensive debate has occurred concerning the definition of a "no option" for revascularization patient. In theory this would be a patient who has exhausted available percutaneous or surgical possibilities for revascularization and would have only amputation as an option if ongoing rest pain or tissue loss cannot be corrected. Given that over 70,000 major amputations occur yearly in the United States, the majority in patients with arterial insufficiency, it would seem that "no option" patients would be abundant in a busy vascular/wound practice. In practice, however, a vascular specialist can almost always attempt some type of percutaneous or surgical option to revascularize a patient unless their medical condition is so poor that the risk would outweigh the benefit of limb salvage. Most patients in this group would not be expected to live long enough to allow enrollment and follow-up in a CLI study requiring a year or so of participation. Unfortunately, many of these percutaneous or surgical procedures performed on CLI patients are "last ditch" attempts after multiple prior interventions have failed and are often associated with limited outcomes. Regardless, vascular specialists have been reluctant to consider patients for a "no option" CLI trial unless all possible options are exhausted leading to an inability to successfully enroll these studies.

In the absence of a better definition of the "no option" patient, CLI studies urgently need other endpoints that can be used to validate the benefit of these potentially valuable therapies. The most likely candidates would be a composite endpoint such as MALE or a similar composite developed using the global rank method as described previously. An endpoint using these methods would allow enrollment of patients who have not exhausted all options for revascularization. If the symptoms do not respond to the clinical trial treatment, whether active or placebo, they may still consider "last ditch" intervention if their condition worsens before amputation is required. These designs are likely to have better appeal to potential subjects as they would have the option to proceed with salvage attempts if necessary thereby facilitating enrollment. To date, composite endpoints have not been accepted by the FDA for late phase clinical trials in cellular therapy.

Interestingly, clinical trials evaluating intravascular devices for the treatment of patients with CLI are typically performed using different endpoints. The development of percutaneous procedures such as intravascular stenting, atherectomy, and drug eluting balloons typically are performed as comparative studies to previously used devices using patency or target lesion revascularization as the primary outcome measures. In these studies, information on amputation and AFS are typically obtained but reported only as secondary outcomes. It is not clear why these invasive therapies associated with potentially life-threatening complications are not held to similar outcome standards by the FDA as those commonly employed for cellular and other angiogenic strategies under development for CLI patients.

SUMMARY

Clinical development of cellular therapies for CLI requires the use of patient-focused trial endpoints that define the benefit of the therapies under study. These endpoints may include amputation, AFS, wound healing, pain scores, QOL scores and surrogate endpoints such as ABI or $TcPO_2$. In early phase studies safety endpoints are primary, while composite endpoints and surrogates are important to determine signal of benefit in trials with limited power. To date Phase-III clinical trials have been held to a primary outcome of amputation or AFS in patients who are not candidates for revascularization leading to difficulty in enrolling patients to complete these studies. It is possible that the development of clinically meaningful composite endpoints or well validated surrogate endpoints will influence clinical trial design and improve our ability to demonstrate the potential clinical benefit of therapies for CLI patients.

REFERENCES

[1] Adam DJ, Beard JD, Cleveland T, Bell J, Bradbury AW, Forbes JF, Fowkes FG, Gillepsie I, Ruckley CV, Raab G, Storkey H. BASIL trial participants. Bypass versus angioplasty in severe ischaemia of the leg (BASIL): multicenter, randomized controlled trial. Lancet 2005;36:1925–34.

[2] Barani J, Nilsson JA, Mattiasson I, Lindblad B, Gottsater A. Inflammatory mediators are associate with 1-year mortality in critical limb ischemia. J Vasc Surg 2005;42:75–80.

[3] Kudo T, Chandra FA, Ahn SS. The effectiveness of percutaneous transluminal angioplasty for the treatement of critical limb ischemia: a 10-year experience. J Vasc Surg 2005;41:423–35.

[4] Bosiers M, Peeters P, Elst FV, Vermassen F, Maleux G, Forneau I, Massin H. Excimer laser assisted angioplasty for critical limb ischemia: results of the LACI Belgium Study. Eur J Vasc Endovasc Surg 2005;29:613–9.

[5] Thomas AR, Raats JW, Lensvelt MM, drGroot HG, Veen EJ, van der Laan L. Conservative treatment in selected patients with critical limb ischemia. World J Surg 2015;39(8):2090–5.

[6] Marston WA, Davies SW, Armstrong B, Farber MA, Mendes RC, Fulton JJ, et al. Natural history of limbs with arterial insufficiency and chronic ulceration treated without revascularization. J Vasc Surg 2006;44:108–14.
[7] Elgzyri T, Larsson J, Thorne J, Eriksson KF, Apelqvist J. Outcome of ischemic foot ulcer in diabetic patients who had no invasive vascular intervention. Eur J Vasc Endovasc Surg 2013;46:110–7.
[8] Brass EP, Anthony R, Dormandy J, Hiatt WR, Jiao J, Nakanishi A, et al. Parenteral therapy with lipo-ecraprost, a lipid-based formulation of a PGE1 analog, does not alter six-month outcomes in patients with critical leg ischemia. J Vasc Surg 2006;43(4):752–9.
[9] Benoit E, O'Donnell TF Jr, Kitsios GD, Iafrati MD. Improved amputation-free survival in unreconstructable critical limb ischemia and implications for clinical trial design and quality measurement. J Vasc Surg 2012;55:781–9.
[10] Nikol S, Baumgartner I, Van Belle E, Diehm C, Visona A, Capogrossi MC, et al. Therapeutic Angiogenesis with intramuscular NV1FGF improves amputation-free survival in patients with critical limb ischemia. Mol Ther 2008;16:972–8.
[11] Belch J, Hiatt WR, Baumgartner I, Driver IV, Nikol S, Norgren L, van Belle E. on behalf of the TAMARIS Committees and Investigators. Effect of fibroblast growth factor NV1FGF on amputation and death: a randomized placebo-controlled trial of gene therapy in critical limb ischaemia. Lancet 2011;377:1929–37.
[12] Vallabhaneni R, Kalbaugh CA, Kouri A, Farber MA, Marston WA. Current accepted hemodynamic criteria for critical limb ischemia do not accurately stratify patients at high risk for limb loss. J Vasc Surg 2014;63(1):105–13.
[13] Powell RJ, Marston WA, Berceli SA, Guzman R, Henry TD, Longcore AT, Stern TP, Watling S, Bartel RL. Cellular therapy with ixmyelocel-T to treat critical limb ischemia: The randomized, double-blind, placebo-controlled RESTORE-CLI trial. Mol Ther 2012;20(6):1280–6.
[14] Iafrati MD, Hallett JW, Geils G, Pearl G, Lumsden A, Peden E, Bandyk D, et al. Early results and lessons learned from a multicenter randomized, double-blind trial of bone marrow aspirate concentrate in critical limb ischemia. J Vasc Surg 2011;54:1650–8.
[15] Treiman GS, Copland S, Yellin AE, Lawrence PF, McNamara RM, Treiman RL. Wound infections involving infrainguinal autogenous vein grafts: a current evaluation of factors determining successful graft preservation. J Vasc Surg 2001;33:948–54.
[16] Marston WA, Hanft J, Norwood P, Pollak R. Dermagraft Diabetic Foot Ulcer Study Group. The efficacy and safety of Dermagraft in improving the healing of chronic diabetic foot ulcers: results of a prospective randomized trial. Diabetes Care 2003;26(6):1701–5.
[17] Veves A, Falanga V, Armstrong DG, et al. Graftskin, a human skin equivalent, is effective in the management of noninfected neuropathic diabetic foot ulcers: a prospective randomized multicenter clinical trial: Apligraf Diabetic Foot Ulcer Study. Diabetes Care 2001;24:290.
[18] Steed DL. Diabetic Ulcer Study Group: clinical evaluation of recombinant human platelet-derived growth factor for the treatment of lower extremity diabeticulcers. J Vasc Surg 1995;21(1):71–8.
[19] Sprengers RW, Teraa M, Moll FL, de Wit GA, van der Graaf Y, Verhaar MC. Quality of life in patients with no-option critical limb ischemia underlines the need for new effective treatment. J Vasc Surg 2010;52:843–9.
[20] Landry GJ, Esmonde NO, Lewis JR, Azarbal AF, Liem TK, Mitchell EL, Moneta GL. Objective measurement of lower extremity function and quality of life after surgical revascularization for critical lower extremity ischemia. J Vasc Surg 2014;60(1):136–42.
[21] Conjin AP, Jens S, Terwee CB, Breek JC, Koelemay MJ. Assessing the quality of available patient reported outcome measures for intermittent claudication: a systematic review using the COSMIN checklist. Eur J Vasc Endovasc Surg 2015;49:316–34.

[22] Hoyer C, Sandermann J, Paludan JP, Pavar S, Petersen LJ. Diagnostic accuracy of laser Doppler flowmetry versus strain gauge plethysmography for segmental pressure measurement. J Vasc Surg 2013;58:1563–70.

[23] Kavros SJ, Delis KT, Turner NS, Voll AE, Liedl DA, Gloviczki P, Rooke TW. Improving limb salvage in critical ischemia with intermittent pneumatic compression: a controlled study with 18-month follow-up. J Vasc Surg 2008;47:543–9.

[24] Yamada T, Ohta T, Ishibashi H, Sugimoto I, Iwata H, Takahashi M, Kawanishi J. Clinical reliability and utility of skin perfusion pressure measurement in ischemic limbs – Comparison with other noninvasive diagnostic methods. J Vasc Surg 2008;47:318–23.

[25] Conte MS, Geraghty PJ, Bradbury AW, Hevelone ND, Lipsitz SR, Moneta GL, Nehler MR, Powell RJ, Sidawy AN. Suggested objective performance goals and clinical trial design for evaluating catheter-based treatment of critical limb ischemia. J Vasc Surg 2009;50:1462–73.

[26] Goodney PP, Schanzer A, DeMartino RR, Nolan BW, Hevelone ND, Conte MS, Powell RJ, Cronenwett JL. Validation of the Society for Vascular Surgery's Objective Performance Goals for critical limb ischemia in everyday vascular surgery practice. J Vasc Surg 2011;54:100–8.

[27] Subherwal S, Anstrom KJ, Jones WS, Felker MG, Misra S, Conte MS, Hiatt WR, Patel MR. Alternative methodologies for evaluation of composite end points in trials of therapies for critical limb ischemia. Am Heart J 2012;164:277–84.

[28] Teraa M, Sprengers RW, Schutgens RE, Slaper-Cortenback IC, van der Graaf Y, Algra A, van der Tweel I, et al. Effect of repetitive intra-arterial infusion of bone marrow mononuclear cells in patients with no-option limb ischemia: the randomized, double-blind, placebo-controlled Rejuvinating Endothelial Progenitor Cells via Transcutaneous Intra-arterial Supplementation (Juventas) trial. Circulation 2015;131:851–60.

[29] Prozchaka V, Gumelec J, Jaluvka F, Salounova D, Lonszta T, Czerny D, Krajca J, et al. Cell therapy, a new standard in management of chronic critical limb ischemia and foot ulcer. Cell Transplant 2010;19:1413–24.

[30] Walter D, Krankenberg H, Balzer JA, Kalka C, Baumgartner I, Schluter M, Tonn T, et al. Intraarterial administration of bone marrow mononuclear cells in patients with critical limb ischemia. A randomized-start, placebo-controlled pilot trial (PROVASA). Circ Cardiovasc Interv 2011;4:26–37.

[31] Kawamoto A, Katayama M, Handa N, Kinoshita M, Takano H, Horii M, Sadamoto K, et al. Intramuscular transplantation of G-CSF-mobilized CD34(+) cells in patients with critical limb ischemia: a phase I/IIa, multicenter, single-blinded, dose-escalation clinical trial. Stem Cells 2009;27:2857–64.

[32] Lasordo DW, Kibbe MR, Mendelsohn F, Marston W, Driver VR, Sharafuddin M, Teodorescu V. A randomized, controlled pilot study of autologous CD34+ cell therapy for critical limb ischemia. Circ Cardiovasc Interv 2012;5:821–30.

[33] Murphy MP, Lawson JH, Rapp BM, Dalsing MC, Klein J, Wilson MG, Hutchins GD, March KL. Autologous bone marrow mononuclear cell therapy is safe and promotes amputation free survival in patients with critical limb ischemia. J Vasc Surg 2011;53:1565–74.

[34] Gupta PK, Chullikana A, Parakh R, Desai S, Das A, Gottipamula S, Krishnamurthy S. A double blind randomized placego controlled phase I/II study assessing the safety and efficacy of allogeneic bone marrow derived mesenchymal stem cell in critical limb ischemia. J Transl Med 2013;11:143.

[35] Lu D, Chen B, Liang Z, Deng W, Jiang Y, Li S, Xu J, et al. Comparison of bone marrow mesenchymal stem cells with bone marrow derived mononuclear cells for treatment of diabetic critical limb ischemia and foot ulcer: a double-blind, randomized, controlled trial. Diabetes Res Clin Pract 2011;92:26–36.

Index

D

E

Q

R

S

FSC
www.fsc.org
MIX
Papier | Fördert
gute Waldnutzung
FSC® C083411

Kolibri 360 GmbH
Ferdinand-Jühlke-Straße 7
99095 Erfurt, Deutschland
produktsicherheit@kolibri360.de

seen in the TiWS group. For group CO, the achievement motive in itself leads to rejecting the idea of founding a business. Thus, they reflect on what they think is required of them and weigh the consequences for their private lives on the identity level. In group CO, structures and symbolic representations in the context of the structural category "gender" have no influence.

14.6 Discussion

In general, the result is to be understood as an exemplary answer to the research question, in which different background factors and their intersections in relation to class, body, race, and gender become clear. In order to verify the groups of intersectional inequalities as typical for students without start-up interest and intention, several more interviews would have to be conducted both within the same study program and across study programs at different universities.

The results show that social inequality or diversity in the context of entrepreneurship education cannot be examined on the basis of a single inequality category such as class or gender in an academic context. The emergence of diversity and its effects must be considered in the context of multiple and, above all, intersecting categories of inequality. In addition to that, following a reflexive understanding of diversity (Bührmann, 2020) leads to a) the necessity of researcher reflections (e. g. the situatedness of the researcher in the research field) and b) the support of knowledge generation regarding relevant dimensions of diversity for equal founding support at universities.

In this case, quantitative studies with an assumed master category, such as gender, would not be able to capture the inequalities of students realistically. The study shows particularly clearly in the group of students who think in worst-case scenarios that disadvantage must be assumed here due to the interconnectedness of gender and race. This is because men and women are influenced by the traditional, patriarchal gender roles of their families of origin with immigration experiences of poverty and thus reject starting their own businesses. Examining the connection and interconnectedness between gender, race, class, and body and how these aspects affect someone's intention to start a business is novel. Therefore, before exploring such a phenomenon quantitatively, different types of connections should be explored qualitatively.

Despite the reflexive approach to diversity within this study, it became clear that students who strive for financial security belong to a group that is not considered in entrepreneurship education, which in this paper is understood as entrepreneurship education to promote new entrepreneurs and start-up companies. In most events, funding, and other formats to raise awareness for the topic of business start-ups in the context of higher education, it is visible that they do not capture and support students of this type. Prejudices are often neither reduced nor is starting one's own business discussed as a possible future form of earning a livelihood. Many students remain unaffected by entrepreneurship education. This finding in the survey testifies to a rather limited perspective of universities on their tasks. Although universities have become more entrepreneurial and support proactive solutions to societal problems (Ferreira et al., 2018), most of them forgot about a diverse and open-minded perspective. Although, different entrepreneurship education concepts that look at awareness raising and qualification exist (Fayolle et al., 2019; Gründungsradar, 2020). However, most of them already assume an existing intention to set up a company (Bijedic, 2019). Future research projects could look at the different entrepreneurship education offers with regard to diversity in order to show possible diversity and corresponding development possibilities for an inclusive offer. Moreover, entrepreneurship education in higher education can be made inclusive in terms of sensitizing students through the results. So that disadvantaged underrepresented groups are also included in the organization of teaching formats of entrepreneurship education.

Furthermore, the study's results also showed that students with a positive role model in starting a business (such as the family entrepreneurship or role model theory; Morgenroth et al., 2015; Bosma et al., 2012a, b) still don't want to start their own business at the time of the survey. Here, values and norms form the framework for refusing to start up one's own business. This is also reflected in the students' narrow view of entrepreneurship, which undermines the positive role model. The performance principle should be mentioned here again, which outweighs a positive role model in the family or a role model who has similarities with the students (Dasgupta, 2011; Ahn et al., 2020). This finding has not yet been taken into account in the role model research discussion. The findings to date consider gender differences and personal relationships/networks (families). First further developments of the role model theory with regard to the study of students with low and high self-esteem (Chen et al., 2016; Lockwood et al., 2002) indicate – like in the work at hand – that the influence of role models is subject to personal factors such as self-esteem or, in this case, the performance principle, and that gender should be considered less specifically as a sole indicator for the selection of role models.

By answering the research question, we have made different contributions to the advancement of the theory of planned behavior or research in the field of founding intention. This is because, with this study and closer examination of its underlying theories, the theory of planned behavior can be developed further. This includes refining the background factors that have so far received little attention. These can now be specified more precisely on the basis of the knowledge gained with the help of the applied research method. These include intersections of class and race. It is relevant to note that there is not one specific category of "gender," as is so often assumed, but intersections of different categories can result in perceived barriers to founding.

The application of intersectionality analysis in entrepreneurship education opened up a new field for the method itself and a methodological enrichment for entrepreneurship education. The method presented here in a transparent and comprehensible way can thus be used in entrepreneurship education research and enrich previous findings, which were predominantly focused only on individual categories.

The authors are aware of the fact that the findings are based on a study that refers to only a few cases. However, this is common in the application of said method. At the same time, this can be seen as a limitation and further cases as well as interviews with students with an affinity for entrepreneurship in other universities and disciplines can be conducted and included. In summary, the world of founding support has many aspects that require closer research and continue to keep this research a worthy pursuit.

Implications for entrepreneurship education practice can also be derived from the results. First, entrepreneurship education at universities should identify all students as a target group for equal start-up support and design awareness-raising measures in line with the target group. This means that different approaches are necessary for different target groups. Second, to ensure equal opportunities for students, entrepreneurship education courses at universities must address topics that deal with social and financial security in start-ups. This specifically means that, for example, possibilities should be discussed that show how the risk and uncertainty can be minimized. Third, the prejudices of the various student groups against starting a business should be addressed and discussed realistically. Additionally, information and offers regarding the social security systems should also be made known in concrete terms.

References

Ahn, J. N., Hu, D., & Vega, M. (2020). "Do as I do, not as I say": Using social learning theory to unpack the impact of role models on students' outcomes in education. *Social and Personality Psychology Compass, 14*(2). https://doi.org/10.1111/spc3.12517

Ajzen, I. (1991). The theory of planned behavior. *Organizational Behavior and Human Decision Processes., 50*(2), 179–211.

Ajzen, I. (2012). Values, attitudes, and behavior. In S. Salzborn (Ed.), *Methods, theories, and empirical applications in the social sciences* (pp. 33–38). Springer VS.

Ajzen, I. (2020). The theory of planned behavior: Frequently asked questions. *Human Behavior and Emerging Technologies, 2*(4), 314–324.

Ajzen, I., & Fishbein, M. (2005). The influence of attitudes on behavior. In B. T. Albarracín (Ed.), *The handbook of attitudes* (pp. 173–221). Erlbaum.

Allen, M. R. (2021). Can entrepreneurship be continued from one generation to the next? The answer to that question can be found in the socialization process. In M. R. Allen & W. B. Gartner (Eds.), *Family entrepreneurship* (pp. 75–83). Palgrave Macmillan.

Altmeier, P. (2019, 03. Dezember). *Bundesministerium für Wirtschaft und Energie*. Von https://www.bmwi.de/Redaktion/DE/Pressemitteilungen/2019/20191203-altmaier-start-ups-sind-motor-des-strukturellen-wandels.html. Zugriff: 21.09.2021 abgerufen.

Aronsson, M. (2004). 'Education matters – But does entrepreneurship education? An interview with David birch. Academy of management learning and education. Entrepreneurship Education, S. 289–292. 3 (3).

Austin, M. J., & Nauta, M. M. (2016). Entrepreneurial role-model exposure, self-efficacy, and women's entrepreneurial intentions. *Journal of Career Development, 43*(3), 260–272. https://doi.org/10.1177/0894845315597475

BarNir, A., Watson, W. E., & Hutchins, H. M. (2011). Mediation and moderated mediation in the relationship among role models, self-efficacy, entrepreneurial career intention, and

gender. *Journal of Applied Social Psychology, 41*(2), 270–297. https://doi.org/10.1111/j.1559-1816.2010.00713
Berger, P. L., & Luckmann, T. (1966). *The social construction of reality*. Anchor Books.
Bijedić, T. (2019). Begriffliche und disziplinäre Genese der Entrepreneurship Education. In T. B. Halbfas (Ed.), *Entrepreneurship education* (pp. 21–40). Springer Gabler.
Bosma, N. S., Wennekers, S. & Amorós, J. (2012a). *Global entrepreneurship monitor 2011 extended global report: Entrepreneurs and entrepreneurial employees across the globe*. Abgerufen am 12. August 2020 von GEM: https://www.gemconsortium.org/file/open?fileId=48326
Bosma, N., Hessels, J., Schutjens, V., van Praag, M., & Verheul, I. (2012b). Entrepreneurship and role models. *Journal of Economic Psychology, 33*(2), 410–424. https://doi.org/10.1016/j.joep.2011.03.004
Breuer, F., Muckel, P., & Dieris, B. (2019). *Reflexive grounded theory*. Springer VS.
Bührmann, A. (2020). *Reflexive Diversitätsforschung*. Opladen.
Butler, J. (1992). Contingent Foundations: Feminism and the Question of "Postmodernism". In: Butler J. & Scott, J.W. (Eds.): *Feminists Theorize the Political*, (pp. 3–21), New York: Routledge.
Chen, N., Ding, G., & Li, W. (2016). Do negative role models increase entrepreneurial intentions? The moderating role of self-esteem. *Basic and Applied Social Psychology, 38*(6), 337–350. https://doi.org/10.1080/01973533.2016.1217223
Crenshaw, K. (2010). Die Intersektion von "Rasse" und Geschlecht demarginalisieren: Eine schwarze feministische Kritik am Antidiskriminierungsrecht der feministischen Theorie und der antirassistischen Politik. In H. Lutz, H. Vivar, M. Teresa, & L. Supik (Eds.), *Fokus Intersektionalität: Bewegung und Verortung eines vielschichtigen Konzepts* (pp. 33–54). VS-Verlag.
Dasgupta, N. (2011). Ingroup experts and peers as social vaccines who inoculate the self-concept: The stereotype inoculation model. *Psychological Inquiry, 22*(4), 231–246. https://doi.org/10.1080/1047840X.2011.607313
Degele, N., & Winker, G. (2017). *Intersektionalität als Mehrebenenanalyse*. Von Technische Universität Hamburg. https://doi.org/10.15480/882.382. Zugriff: 02.02.2020 abgerufen.
Dyer, W. G. (2021). Family capital: The key to entrepreneurial and family success. In M. R. Allen & W. B. Gartner (Eds.), *Family entrepreneurship* (pp. 7–21). Palgrave Macmillan.
Dyer, W. G., & Handler, W. (1994). Entrepreneurship and family business: Exploring the connections. *Entrepreneurship Theory and Practice*, 71–83.
Fayolle, A. (2013). Personal views on the future of entrepreneurship education, *Entrepreneurship & Regional Development, 25:7–8*, 692–701, https://doi.org/10.1080/08985626.2013.821318
Fayolle, A., & Linán, F. (2014). The future of research on entrepreneurial intention. *Journal of Business Research, 67*(5), 663–666.
Fayolle, A., Kariv, D., & Matlay, H. (2019). *The role and impact of entrepreneurship education. Methods, teachers and innovative programmes*. Edward Elgar Publishing Limited.
Fellnhofer, K., & Mueller, S. (2018). "I want to be like you!": The influence of role models on entrepreneurial intention. *Journal of Enterprising Culture, 26*(02), 113–153. https://doi.org/10.1142/S021849581850005
Fenstermaker, S., & West, C. (2002). *Doing Gender, Doing Difference*. Routledge.
Ferreira, J. J., Fayolle, A., Ratten, V., & Raposo, M. (2018). The role of entrepreneurial universities in society. In J. J. Ferreira, A. Fayolle, V. Ratten, & M. Raposo (Eds.), *Entrepreneurial Universities* (pp. 1–13). Elgaronline.
Foucault, M. (1977). *Der Wille zum Wissen*. Frankfurt am Main: Suhrkamp.
Ganz, K., & Hausotter, J. (2020). *Intersektionale Sozialforschung*. Transcript Verlag.
Geldof, D. (2016). *Superdiversity in the heart of Europe. How migration changes our society*. acco.
Glaser, B. & Strauss, A. (1998). Grounded Theory. Strategien qualitativer Forschung. Göttingen: Hans Huber. [Orig. 1967].
Gründungsradar. (2020). *Gründungssensibilisierung und Gründungsqualifizierung an Hochschulen*. Von Gründungsradar: https://www.gruendungsradar.de/bausteine/gruendungs-sensibilisierung-2020. Zugriff: 13.10.21. abgerufen.

Halbfas, B. G. (2006). Entrepreneurship Education an Hochschulen. Eine wirtschaftspädagogische und - didaktische Analyse. Paderborn: Eusl.
Hindle, K. (2007). Teaching entrepreneurship at university: From the wrong building to the right philosophy. In A. Fayolle & D. Redford (Eds.), *Handbook of research in entrepreneurship education* (A general perspective) (Vol. 1, pp. 104–125). Edward Elgar Publishing Limited.
Hofmann, R. (2012). Gesellschaftstheoretische Grundlagen für einen reflexiven und inklusiven Umgang mit Diversitäten in Organisationen. In R. H.-E. Bendl (Ed.), *Diversität und Diversitätsmanagement* (pp. 23–60). facultas.
Högsdal, N., Münch, J., & Bauer, H. (2020). *Entrepreneurship meets Education – Förderung der Gründungskultur an Hochschulen.* Von Hochschule Reutlingen: https://publikationen.reutlingen-university.de/frontdoor/deliver/index/docId/2944/file/2944.pdf. Zugriff: 04.09.21 abgerufen.
Johannisson, B. (2018). Limits to and prospects of entrepreneurship education in the academic context. In A. Fayolle (Ed.), *A research agenda for entrepreneurship education* (pp. 139–163). Edward Elgar Publishing.
Jungbauer-Gans, M., & Gottburgsen, A. (2021). *Migration, Mobilität und soziale Ungleichheit in der Hochschulbildung*. Springer VS.
Karimi, S., Biemans, J. A., & H., Lans, T., Chizari, M., & Mulder, M. (2014). Effects of role models and gender on students' entrepreneurial intentions. *European Journal of Training and Development, 38*(8), 694–727. https://doi.org/10.1108/EJTD-03-2013-0036
Knapp, G.-A. (2005). "Intersectionality" – ein neues Paradigma feministischer Theorie? Zur transatlantischen Reise von "race, class, gender". *Feministische Studien, 1*, 68–82.
Krell, G., & Sieben, B. (2011). Diversity Management: Chancengleichheit für alle und auch als Wettbewerbsvorteil. In G. O. Krell (Ed.), *Chancengleichheit durch Personalpolitik* (pp. 155–174). Gabler.
Lange, A. (2012). *Subjektive gründungsbezogene Überzeugungen Studierender*. Optimus.
Laspita, S., Breugst, N., Heblich, S., & Patzelt, H. (2012). Intergenerational transmission of entrepreneurial intentions. *Journal of Business Venturing, 27*(4), 414–435. https://doi.org/10.1016/j.jbusvent.2011.11.006
Leontiy, H., & Schulz, M. (2020). Die Vielfältigkeit der Diversität – Eine Einführung. In I. H. Leontiy, M. Schulz, & Ethnographie und Diversität. (Eds.), *Wissensproduktion an den Grenzen und die Grenzen der Wissensproduktion* (pp. 1–23). Springer VS.
Linán, F., & Fayolle, A. (2015). A systematic literature review on entrepreneurial intentions: Citation, thematic analyses, and research agenda. *International Entrepreneurship and Management Journal, 11*(4), 907–933.
Lockwood, P., Jordan, C. H., & Kunda, Z. (2002). Motivation by positive or negative role models: Regulatory focus determines who will best inspire us. *Journal of Personality and Social Psychology, 83*(4), 854–864. https://doi.org/10.1037//0022-3514.83.4.854
Lutz, H. (2001). Differenz als Rechenufgabe: Über die Relevanz der Kategorien Race, Class, Gender. In I. H. Lutz & N. Wenning (Eds.), *Unterschiedlich verschieden* (pp. 215–230). Opladen.
Martinez, A., & Agwunobi, A. J. (2018). Intersectionality and mixed methods for social context in entrepreneurship. *International Journal of Entrepreneurial Behavior & Research*. https://doi.org/10.1108/IJEBR-12-2017-0498. Abgerufen am 15. August 2020.
McCall, L. (2005). The Complexity of Intersectionality (T. U. Press, Hrsg.). *Signs* (Vol. 30, No. 3), S. 1771–1800.
McMullan, E., & Long, W. A. (1987). Entrepreneurship education in the nineties. *Journal of Business Venturing, 2*, 261–275.
Metzger, G. (2015). *KfW research*. Abgerufen am 27. August 2020 von Deutschland einig Gründerland? Mitnichten!: https://www.kfw.de/PDF/Download-Center/Konzernthemen/Research/PDF-Dokumente-Fokus-Volkswirtschaft/Fokus-Nr.-111-November-2015-Deutschland-einig-Gr%C3%BCnderland.pdf
Morgenroth, T., Ryan, M. K., & Peters, K. (2015). The motivational theory of role modeling: How role models influence role aspirants' goals. *Review of General Psychology, 19*(4), 465–483. https://doi.org/10.1037/gpr0000059

Pablo-Lerchundi, I., Morales-Alonso, G., & González-Tirados, R. M. (2015). Influences of parental occupation on occupational choices and professional values. *Journal of Business Research, 68*(7), 1645–1649. https://doi.org/10.1016/j.jbusres.2015.02.011

Radu, M., & Loué, C. (2008). Motivational impact of role models as moderated by "ideal" vs. "ought self-guides" identifications. *Journal of Enterprising Culture, 16*(4), 441–465. https://doi.org/10.1142/S0218495808000223

Sarasvathy, S. D. (2008). *Effectuation: Elements of entrepreneurial expertise*. Edward Elgar.

Shapero, A. (1982). Social dimensions of entrepreneurship. In D. L. C. A. Kent (Ed.), *Encyclopedia of entrepreneurship* (pp. 72–90). Prentice Hall.

Shapero, A. (1984). *The entrepreneurial event*. Lexington Books.

The Combahee River Collective. (1982). A black feminist statement. In G. Hull (Ed.), *All the women are white, all the blacks are men, but some of us are brave* (pp. 13–22). Feminist Press.

Torrens, E., & Barahona, A. (2012). Why are some evolutionary trees in natural history museums prone to being misinterpreted? Evolution Education and Outreach. Vol. 5, Nr. 1, S. 76–100.

Van Auken, H., Fry, F. L., & Stephens, P. (2006). The influence of role models on entrepreneurial intentions. *Journal of Developmental Entrepreneurship, 11*(2), 157–167. https://doi.org/10.1142/S1084946706000349

Vedder, G. (2009). Diversity Management: Grundlagen und Entwicklung im internationalen Vergleich. In S. K. Andresen (Ed.), *Gender und Diversity: Albtraum oder Traumpaar? Interdisziplinärer Dialog zur "Modernisierung" von Geschlechter- und Gleichstellungspolitik* (pp. 111–132). VS Verlag für Sozialwissenschaften.

Walter, S. G. (2008). *Gründungsintention von Akademikern*. Gabler.

Winker, G., & Degele, N. (2010). *Intersektionalität. Zur Analyse sozialer Ungleichheit*. transcript.

Winker, G., & Degele, N. (2011). Intersectionality as multi-level analysis: Dealing with social inequality. *European Journal of Women's Studies., 18*(1), 51–66.

www.ingramcontent.com/pod-product-compliance
Ingram Content Group UK Ltd.
Pitfield, Milton Keynes, MK11 3LW, UK
UKHW020810290926
15470UKWH00003B/1068
* 9 7 8 3 0 3 1 5 0 1 6 3 0 *

www.ingramcontent.com/pod-product-compliance
Ingram Content Group UK Ltd.
Pitfield, Milton Keynes, MK11 3LW, UK
UKHW020810290926
15470UKWH00003B/1068
* 9 7 8 3 0 3 1 5 0 1 6 3 0 *